SITE SAFETY HANDBOOK FOR THE PETROLEUM INDUSTRY

SITE SAFETY HANDBOOK FOR THE PETROLEUM INDUSTRY

Chidi Venantius Efobi

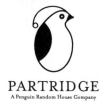

PARTRIDGE
A Penguin Random House Company

To order additional copies of this book, contact
Toll Free 800 101 2657 (Singapore)
Toll Free 1 800 81 7340 (Malaysia)
orders.singapore@partridgepublishing.com

www.partridgepublishing.com/singapore

Contents

Dedicated to

God Almighty, for His grace and favors;

Ezioma, my amiable wife, for her love, affection, understanding and patience;

Chimazuru and Chizitere, our children, for their affection and warmth;

Ferdinand, my daddy, for being a real dad and teaching me the basic art of writing;

Celine, my late mum, for being a real mum and teaching me to be disciplined;

Uncle Arthur Aso, for inspiring me to be an engineer.

<u>Warning</u>

The safety measures stated in this book are just generic guidelines and should not be taken as standards. It does not remove the liability from the reader to use sound engineering practice and established standards to make judgments in specific situations he/she encounters.

Chapter 1

OVERVIEW OF THE PETROLEUM INDUSTRY

The petroleum industry consists of exploration, extraction, separation/ processing, refining, transportation and marketing of crude oil and petroleum products. It is usually divided into upstream, midstream and downstream sectors.

The upstream sector, sometimes referred to as the exploration and production (E&P), explores and extracts crude oil and natural gas from the earth's crust.

The midstream sector separates, processes, transports, stores, and markets crude oil, natural gas, natural gas liquids and other useful derivatives (like sulphur).

The downstream sector consists of oil refineries, petrochemical plants, petroleum products tank farms, gas distribution companies, gas stations etc. The downstream sector provides products such as gasoline, diesel, kerosene, jet-fuel, heating oil, asphalt, lube oil, fertilizers, plastics, synthetic rubber, pharmaceuticals, pesticides, natural gas etc. to the final consumers

1.1 Exploration

The search for petroleum (known as exploration) most times takes workers to remote locations such as dense forests, deserts, swamps and off shores and starts with aerial surveys and surface observation by geologists and geophysicists. When these professionals see the kind of the rock formations that might contain petroleum, they conduct seismic surveys that give better understanding of the underground rock formations.

During a seismic survey, lines of sensitive receivers, known as geophones, are laid on the ground. Explosions or mechanical vibrations are then created on the surface and the geophones record the energy reflected back as seismic waves from rock layers. The recorded data are then processed and it gives a picture of the sedimentary structures in the earth's crust at the specific location. Geologists and geophysicist have the training to look at these pictures and determine the location and extent of porous layers that have the potential of being suitable traps for petroleum.

1.2 Drilling

After the potential locations of petroleum traps are determined, deep holes are punched to them in order to be certain whether or not they contain sufficient and commercially viable oil or gas quantities. This process of holes punching is referred to as drilling and they are conducted with equipment know as rigs. There are various types and sizes of drilling rigs. The types that are used on land are constituted of different components that are assembled and taken apart in sections for ease of movement between locations. They are usually moved from one location to another on road trailers and this process is called rig move.

Drilling basically involves revolving steel bit (usually studded with industrial diamonds or tungsten carbide) at the bottom of a string of pipe that grinds a hole through the rock layers into the earth's crust. As the bit drills deeper, additional pipes are threaded onto the top of the string. Rotary table on the rig floor rotates the drill string on some land rigs. On offshore and other land rigs, hydraulic or electric motors suspended above the rig floor drive the drill strings. These are called top drives. Some computers help to guide the string to the specific location that has the potential of containing petroleum.

As the drilling is going on, fluid called drilling mud lubricates the bit, removes rock cuttings, and stabilizes the pressure in the hole. The mud can be a suspension of chemicals and minerals in either water or oil. The former are called water based and the latter, oil based mud. During drilling the mud is pumped down the hole through the drill pipe and it circulates back to the surface through the space outside the pipe, known as the annulus. The embedded cuttings are then removed by a vibrating screen known as the shale shaker and the mud, re-circulated. Sometimes wells are drilled without mud, may be to increase penetration or avoid contaminating sensitive rock formations with water or oil. In such instances, compressed air is used to remove the cuttings.

Drilling of wells is conducted in stages, beginning with a surface hole drilled to reach a depth between 60 and 400 meters, depending on the design. When the surface hole is completed, the drill string is pulled out and steel pipes, known as surface casing, are inserted and cemented in place. The surface casing serves three key purposes, viz:it prevents wall collapse, controls the flow of mud and prevents the contamination of groundwater aquifers.

When the surface casing is in place, the blowout preventer (BOP) system is installed on the top of it, below the rig floor. BOPs, as the name implies, are simply large valves that help to prevent blowout, which is an uncontrolled gushing out of formation fluid (crude oil and gas). It does this by either sealing off the annulus or shearing of the drill pipe and sealing of the hole entirely. The use of this system, however, comes as a secondary resort. Formation fluid is primarily held in check by varying the density of the drilling mud. If these barriers fail and a blowout takes place, it could lead to disastrous consequences, including complete loss of the rig and/or multiple fatalities.

Extreme care is taken when drilling wells that have the potential to contain hydrogen sulfide (sour gas) because loss of containment could affect not only the workers on the rig site but also nearby residents. Before the commencement of such drilling activities, effective emergency response planning, public consultation, provision of relevant safety equipment and training of workers for sour gas operations should be carried out. In some instances, the emergency response preparedness could include giving authorization to the rig superintendent to set the rig on fire (if there is a blowout) to prevent the spread of the sour gas.

As the drilling progresses, samples of the rock cuttings are taken with the use of coring bits and from the drilling mud (before re-circulation). These samples are examined to understand the age, chemical composition, porosity, permeability, other physical characteristics of the rock and any fluids contained within its formations. Various logs are plotted of these data vis-a-vis the depths/locations from which the samples are taken. Geologists and geophysicists study these logs to determine the quantity of petroleum in place and the best way to efficiently extract them. Sometimes, data is obtained by lowering instruments called logging tools into the well bore to record and transmit information about the formation. These logging instruments can also be installed close to the bit to send data continuously during drilling. There are also various other methods (e.g. drill stem test) of determining the potential of a well.

If all these methods are used and the well indicates to be dry(meaning it is not capable of producing commercial quantities of oil and gas)it is plugged with cement and further activities stopped.

Figure 1: Land Oil Drilling Rig

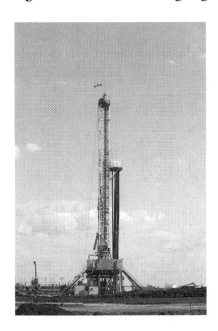

1.3 Completion

If, however, a well is drilled and various studies indicate that it holds commercial quantity of recoverable petroleum, the next stage will be what is called well completion. This is the procedure by which installations are put on a well to enable it to produce safely. The commencement of this procedure involves the installation of production casing. Casings are tubular steel pipes connected by threads and couplings. They are installed the total length of the well bore and have three key functions, viz: ensure safe control of production; prevent water ingress and rock formations collapsing into the well bore. Once the casings are cemented successfully, the main drilling rig is usually moved away to another location.

When the main drilling rig is moved away, a smaller one is moved in for the installation of the production tubing. These are steel pipes smaller in diameter than the production casing. They are lowered into the casing and held in place with packers. The wellhead (often called Christmas tree) is then installed at the surface end of the string of production tubing. The wellhead consists of valves, chokes and pressure gauges that help to regulate production from the well.

After the production tubing and wellhead are installed, the well is perforated. A perforating gun (laden with explosive charges) is lowered into the well on an electrical wireline to a specified depth; an electrical impulse is then triggered to fire the charges to perforate the casing, surrounding cement and formation rock. This enables the formation fluid (crude oil and gas) to flow into the casing, the production tubing and finally to the surface through the well head.

The pressure in some wells is sufficient to push the oil to the surface and others require artificial lift. There are several types of artificial lift, one of which is known as gas lift. This involves sending compressed gas into formation through a pre-installed gas lift mandrels on the production tubing. The compressed gas enhances the flow of the crude oil to the surface by boosting the pressure. Another type of artificial lift involves lowering a pump down the tubing to the bottom of the well on a string of steel rods, known as the rod string. The rod string is connected to an electric motor that powers the pump. Some of these types of pumps are the 'nodding donkeys' popular in many oil fields in the United States of America.

In some oil and gas wells, some kind of physical or chemical stimulation is carried out on the formation to enable the hydrocarbons move more easily to the well bore. One common method of stimulation is known as acidizing. This involves the injection of acids under pressure into the formation via the producing tubing and perforations. These acids dissolve some portions of the formation rock, thereby creating channels for oil to flow more easily into the well bore Another common method of stimulation is known as fracking. It involves fluid like water or oil product being pumped down the well under pressure that creates some kind of cracks in the formation. Hard particles (e.g. glass beads, aluminum pellets, and sand) are pumped with the fluid. These particles hold open the cracks thereby enabling hydrocarbons to flow out more easily to the well bore. The discovery of fracking has revolutionized the oil industry as fluids hitherto thought to be irrecoverable are now being recovered.

Figure 2: Crude Oil Pumps

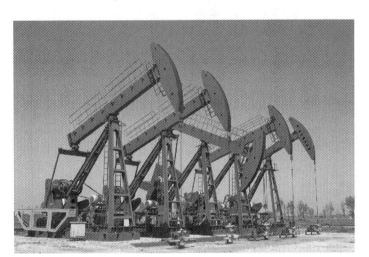

1.4 Transportation

Fluids that are produced from the well bore are a mixture of hydrocarbons, water, sand, hydrogen sulfide and other impurities at high pressure and temperature. Petroleum fluid in this state will require to be treated, separated and processed to meet customer specifications. Separation and processing facilities are expensive and would make no economic sense if located close to individual wells. Hence hydrocarbon fluids will require being transported and gathered into some central processing facilities. Pipelines networks are the most cost effective method of transportation of hydrocarbon fluids but road and rail tankers are sometimes used.

1.5 Separation& Processing

The first stage in the processing of hydrocarbon fluids takes place in a separation plant. In a typical gas and oil separation plant (GOSP), the hydrocarbons are gathered and sent to the separator vessels. The vessels operate close to atmospheric pressure hence when high pressure hydrocarbon fluids are passed into them the gaseous elements are flashed into an overhead pipeline. From there, they are either sent out for further processing in a gas plant or to be flared. The liquid element undergoes further processing to reduce the water and salt content. When the liquid stabilizes, the unwanted solids (e.g.

sand) settle at the bottom of the separator. The crude oil is skimmed off and pumped to refineries or terminals (through pipelines) for shipment overseas.

The gaseous elements taken off at the separators for further processing are compressed, cooled, dehydrated, much of the hydrogen sulfide removed and piped to various customers. If they need to be shipped to large distant customers they are liquefied prior to shipment and this is done in facilities known as liquefied natural gas plants. For gases that are rich in ethane, propane, butane and other heavier hydrocarbons, these are recovered as condensate hydrocarbons from the gas. The recovery process is carried out in natural gas liquid plants.

It is worthy of note that hydrocarbon gases can either come out from the well in solution of crude oil and when the pressure is reduced in GOSP separators, the gases flash out of the solution. This type is called associated gas. On the other hand, there are wells that produce only gases. These gases that are produced from exclusive gas wells are called non-associated gases.

Hydrocarbon gases are used for power generation, heating purposes and feedstock (raw material) in petrochemical and pharmaceutical industries.

Figure 3: Gas and Oil Separation Plant

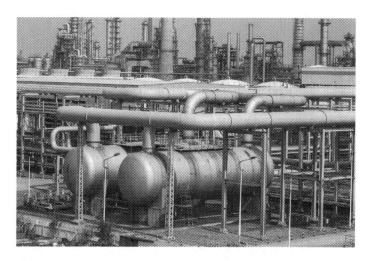

1.6 Refining

Crude oil consists mainly of hydrocarbons. Refining is simply the chemical process of breaking up and sometimes re-linking of the hydrocarbon chains to produce desired products. In addition, undesirable constituents of the hydrocarbon fluid (such as sulfur, nitrogen, oxygen, water and other trace elements) are removed and disposed-off safely.

The refining process involves heating the hydrocarbon fluid to about 350° Celsius and then pumping it into a fractionating tower. At that temperature, the oil vaporizes and rises up the tower through trays with holes in them. As the gas cools, it starts coming down from the top. As it does so the different components condense back into several distinct liquids at different levels of the tower. Lighter liquids (e.g. gasoline and kerosene) condense nearer the top of the tower, while heavier ones (e.g. lubricants and waxes) condense nearer the bottom.

In addition, reforming, alkylation and cracking processes are also used in the refineries to "rearrange" some hydrocarbon components into better commercially desirable ones.

The final products from the refineries are transported either via pipelines or trucks to various distribution posts and customers.

Chapter 2

GENERAL SAFETY

2.1 Hazard Identification, Risk Assessment and Risk Control

Preamble– The petroleum industry is full of materials, activities and processes that have potential to cause harm to people, property or the environment. These are called hazards. Hazards should be proactively managed to prevent them from resulting into accidents.

An accident is an unpleasant, unexpected, unforeseen, or unintended happening that results in harm to people, damage to property, environment or company reputation.

In the petroleum industry a businesslike approach to management of hazards in the workplace should be employed. This approach is called safety management system. It provides a systematic way to pro-actively identify hazards, assess the risks and put controls in place while maintaining assurance that these risk controls are effective. A good safety management system is woven around tasks/activities of the normal business processes and becomes part of the way work is done.

In a simplistic manner, identifying hazards is just spotting what can wrong. Assessing the risk is evaluating how bad it could be (consequence or severity) and how often it might happen (likelihood or frequency). Assessing risk enables management to prioritize mitigation measures. More resources are likely to be deployed towards mitigating higher risk hazards than lower ones.

Consequences in safety management denote the undesirable effects of an accident. A good safety management system pro-actively assesses all the effects of an accident and puts measures in place to prevent situations from degenerating. For an example, if there is a car crash, the probability of death (or serious harm) will depend on whether or not the occupants have their seat belts and how quickly they are rescued and given medical attention.

Likelihood denotes how often the accident has taken place (from objective records) either in the facility, company, country or industry. For example, it is more likely that hydrogen sulfide will be released and kill workers in a drill site than aero plane falling from the sky onto the rig. Hence hydrogen sulfide is a higher risk and more resources should be deployed to put control and recovery measures in place for hydrogen sulfide release than planes falling from the sky.

Controls are measures put in place to prevent a hazard resulting into an accident. Recovery measures prevent the effect of an accident getting worse.

Hazard Identification – Hazard identification is the first step of risk assessment. It is the duty of every personnel that works in the petroleum industry to constantly look out for hazards in the workplace and report them to their supervisors. However, in a formal setting, hazard identification is conducted by a team of personnel competent and experienced in the work process, materials and activities. There are various methods of systematically identifying hazards to ensure that nothing is left and these are: tour of the work area and speaking to the workforce; manufacturers' handbooks; material safety data sheets; labels on materials/equipment; approved codes of practice; industrial standards; generic hazard list; incidents or ill-health records; safety inspection/audit reports; and experience of the team.

Persons at risk – At job sites, regular employees and full-time contractors are the most persons at risk and hence, it is important to ensure that they are competent to perform the jobs they are assigned. However, it is equally important that other groups of person who spend time in or around the workplace be identified (e.g. young or newly employed workers, trainees, visitors, irregular contractors and the public). The risk assessment should include any additional controls required due to the vulnerability of any of these groups.

Evaluation of risk level – Risk level is simply a product of the likelihood or frequency of occurrence and the severity or consequence of harm. A credible evaluation criterion should be pre-determined before the commencement of the exercise. Most companies use what is called the risk assessment matrix with criteria varying from company to company. Figures 3,4& 5 are examples of criteria used in risk evaluation.

Figure 4: Example of Likelihood/Frequency criteria

Level	Description
1	Very low: Never heard of in the industry
2	Low: Some incidents have been reported in the industry
3	Medium: Incident has occurred in the company
4	High: Incident has occurred severally in the company.

Figure 5: Example of Severity/Consequence Criteria

Level	Description
1	Very low: No injury or health effect
2	Low: Minor injury or minor health effect, requiring just a first aid treatment.
3	Medium: Serious injury or serious health effect resulting in lost workdays
4	High: Fatality or permanent total disability

Figure 6: Example of a Risk Matrix

LIKELIHOOD					
	4				VERY HIGH RISK
	3			HIGH RISK	
	2		MEDIUM RISK		
	1	LOW RISK			
		1	2	3	4
		CONSEQUENCE			

Risk Control Measures – Having assessed the risk, the next step will be to put measures in place to prevent them from harming people, environment or property. In determining what measure to adopt, the following are the hierarchy of controls, in order of effectiveness;

✓ Elimination& Substitution

These are the most effective methods of avoiding a hazard and its associated risk. Elimination is when a process or activity is totally eliminated or abandoned because the associated risk is too high for the expected benefit. Substitution is the use of less hazardous form of a material or substance. An example is the substitution of asbestos pipes for carrying drinking water with PVC pipes.

✓ Engineering controls

This is the control of risks by means of engineering design rather than preventive action by workers. There are several methods of achieving such controls and some of these are: controlling the risk at the source (for example, the use of dust filters); isolating the equipment with guard, barrier or enclosure; insulating electrical or extreme temperature hazards; ventilating away the hazardous atmosphere.

✓ Administrative Controls

There are various administrative controls, such as changing work methods/ patterns (changing methods of conducting an activity to reduce or eliminate exposure to harmful substances); good housekeeping (keeping the work place clean and tidy at all times and maintaining good storage systems for hazardous substances); safe systems of work (safe method of performing activities, normally written and communicated to personnel via training); training and information.

✓ Personal protective equipment

Personal protective equipment (PPE) is the last line of defense and should only be used as a last resort. This will be discussed in greater detail in section 2.3.

2.2 Risk Assessment Tools

There are several risk assessment tools and methodologies available. The choice of tool will depend on type of activity and equipment, number of workers, particular features of the workplace or process and any specific risks.

Job Safety Analysis (JSA) – this is sometimes referred to as Job Hazard Analysis (JHA) or Task Hazard Analysis (THA). JSA should be the most basic risk assessment tool for any non-routine or potentially hazardous activity in the petroleum industry. It is simply looking at the work task and considering what is the safest way to complete it. It is a method of gaining awareness of the hazards involved in completing the task and proactively taking action to prevent an injury.

The following are the steps to conduct a JSA.

- Constitute a JSA team, which should be those involved in the activity.
- Write down the tasks that make up the activity, step by step.
- For each step, identify the hazards of the task and the environment.
- For each identified hazard, evaluate the risk, identify who could be harmed, and list the measures (control and recovery) that need to be put in place to eliminate or minimize the risk.
- For each control or recovery measure, identify who is responsible for implementation.
- It is advisable to document JSA in a tabular format(a column each for job step, hazards, risk, persons at risk, control/recovery measures and responsible party).
- JSA should be well documented, reviewed and approved by supervisory personnel with authority to ensure that all required resources are provided.
- The approved JSA should be communicated to all personnel involved in the activity during a pre-job meeting which must be conducted.
- As the job progresses, adequate supervision should be in place to ensure the documented process is being followed.
- The JSA should be reviewed whenever a documented activity changes, when there is a change of personnel or after an appropriate length of time.

Figure 7: Sample of JSA Table

S/N	Job Steps	Hazards	Likelihood	Consequence	Risk	Control/Recovery Measures	Responsible Party

HAZID (HAZardIDentification) Exercise – HAZID is the first step in primary risk assessment for a new facility. It is a high level review of potential hazards. It uses checklists of hazards to pinpoint material, system, process and facility characteristics that could produce undesirable consequences through the occurrence of an incident. Possible means of eliminating the hazards or controlling the risk are usually identified. It is worthy of note that early identification and assessment of hazards is critical in project decisions at a time when design changes can still be done with minimal cost implication.

Hazard and Operability (HAZOP) Studies – This is a structured and systematic examination of a planned or existing process/facility or operation in order to identify and evaluate problems that may present risk to personnel, equipment or environment. It should also identify problems that may prevent efficient operation. It is conducted by multi-disciplinary team of very experienced professionals and uses standard guide words. The output of HAZOP is as good as the team and so it is important that people who take part in it should be competent in their various fields and have undergone some basic training in HAZOP studies.

Others – There are several other specialized or more detailed tools such as Fire Risk Assessment, Bow-ties, Failure Mode and Effects Analysis, Fire and Explosion Risk Assessment etc.

2.3 Personal Protective Equipment (PPE)

In hazardous work locations, after substitution/elimination, engineering and administrative controls, PPE is the last wall of defense in protecting personnel from hazards. Workers should be trained on how to inspect, use, maintain and store PPEs.

Head Protection –Hard hats should always be worn wherever there are overhead objects, materials or activities that can result in objects falling and when activities being performed can result to electrical shock or burns to the head. This includes construction sites, live plants and other designated areas.

Hard hats should as a minimum have a shell and suspension cradle. Name of manufacturer, date of manufacture, ANSI Z89.1 compliance and class must be written inside a good hard hat. As a rule, they should be replaced five years after the date of manufacture. In addition, the suspension cradle should be replaced every year.

Hard hats that are cracked or have had heavy impact must not be used again but be thrown away. They shall not be painted or have large stickers on them as these tend to hide cracks. Drilling holes in a hard hat weakens it and must not be permitted. To avoid risk of electrocution, metallic hats should not be used when working close to energized electrical equipment.

Eye and Face Protection – Eye protection in form of safety glasses should be worn while performing work where the risks of flying objects entering into workers eyes exist. Where work is being done with chemicals, suitable eye/face protection should be used for protection against chemical splashes. As a rule in the petroleum industry, approved safety glasses should be worn in exploration, drilling, construction and producing sites. This is because pressure hazards exist in most of the locations and loss of containment could send particles flying at high speed. In addition, for personnel performing welding activities approved welder's helmet with the proper lens shade should be worn.

Foot Protection – Safety footwear with leather uppers, and steel toes should be worn at all times in all work locations in the petroleum industry. This is to protect the foot from falling objects, striking against things and piercing by sharp objects. Special types of safety footwear should be worn by workers performing electrical jobs and using jack hammers.

Hand Protection – Suitable gloves should be worn to protect hand from cuts, abrasion, chemicals, extreme temperatures (heat or cold) and electricity. However, they should not be worn in close proximity to moving/rotating equipment in order to prevent being caught between moving parts.

Body Protection – Body covering should be selected and used based on the hazard. Fire retardant clothing should be worn by personnel in locations assessed as having potential for flash fires. Electric arc flash, abrasive blasting, welding, and chemical handling each have body protection suitable for it.

Hearing Protection – Ear defenders should be worn in high noise areas or while performing activities that generate high noise. Workers should never be exposed to noise levels above 85 decibels (dBA) without adequate protection.

Respiratory Protection Equipment (RPE)–These should be worn by personnel exposed to air contaminants above permissible threshold values. The specific type shall depend on the types of contaminants. It is noteworthy that RPE shall be appropriately chosen and personnel who wear them well trained in the inspection, usage and storage. Workers must be closely supervised by experienced personnel while using RPE.

Personal Floatation Device (PFD) - Personal flotation devices (PFDs) are life jackets, life vests, cork jacket, buoyancy aid or flotation suit that are designed to be worn by personnel working above or near water. They assist the wearer, conscious or unconscious, to keep afloat until rescued.

2.4 Emergency Response Planning

An emergency is an unforeseen situation that threatens employees, the public, disrupts or shuts down operations or causes physical or environmental damage. Emergencies may be natural or manmade and include the following:

- Fires/explosions
- Oil/chemical Spill
- Gas release
- Radiological accidents
- Attack by wild animals
- Security or civil disturbances
- Hurricanes/tornadoes/cyclones
- Floods
- Medical
- Man overboard

Every workplace needs a plan for emergencies as they can strike at any time when workers least expect them. The best way to ensure that people and properties are protected is to expect the unexpected and develop a well-thought out emergency response plan to guide personnel when immediate action is necessary. Few people have the ability to think clearly and logically in an emergency so it is important to proactively plan for them.

Brainstorm Credible Scenarios – Planning for emergency starts with forming a team to brainstorm credible scenarios. To do this successfully, a risk assessment of the work or activity should have been conducted. From the risk assessment, it should be determined what, if any, hazards in the workplace could cause an emergency. When the potential emergencies have been identified, the next step is to consider how to respond.

Develop emergency action plan – this includes actions that management and personnel should take to minimize the impact of an emergency. The emergency action plan should include the following:

- Required resources (human and material, on-site and off-site) for tackling identified scenarios; for off-site resources, the location where they are available should be identified;in addition, coordination is required with organizations where off-site resources are located to ensure that they will be readily available when and as required;

- Emergency response organization chart – this chart should clearly show the reporting protocols in an emergency; assigning responsibilities to all key personnel. Technical supports for each type of emergency situation should also be part of this chart;
- Specific procedures to follow for respective emergencies;
- Emergency escape procedures and route assignments, such as floor plans, workplace maps and safe or refuge areas;
- Names, titles, departments and telephone numbers of individuals to contact for additional help (these individuals may be within or outside your organization);
- Procedures for employees, who remain to perform or shut down critical plant operations, operate fire extinguishers or perform other essential services;
- Rescue and medical duties for those designated;
- Means of alerting workers, such as visual and audio alarms;
- Emergency communication systems such as public address system, portable radios, telephones;
- Alternative sources of power supplies for essential equipment;
- A system for accounting for personnel following an evacuation;
- Required training for all response/ support personnel and training schedule;
- Emergency drill schedule.

The plan should be reviewed and approved by company executive with sufficient authority to commit the resources required. The approval and commitment should include timelines for the completion of each required action.

Implement action plan– This includes the following:

- Communication of the plan to all personnel-important information like procedures to follow, key telephone numbers, escape routes/safe areas, and alarm types should be prominently displayed on notice boards and given to all personnel as pocket cards;

- Training all response/support personnel;
- Provision of identified resources (on-site and off-site) and having in place a process of regularly checking and testing them to ensure they are fit for purpose;
- For resources that are identified to be provided by third parties, ensuring that contractual or mutual cooperation agreement are knitted up properly;
- Implementing the approved emergency drill schedule-at the end of each exercise, hold a critique meeting with the key personnel to assess what worked well and what did not;for things that did not work well, initiate action items to ensure that deficiencies are addressed timely.

2.5 Incident Reporting and Investigation

Every organization should have a process put in place to report accidents, incidents or near-misses for immediate action and investigation. The organization needs to identify what needs to be reported, to whom it is to be reported and how to report it, and then put this process into a written procedure.

For example: *Any accident, incident, or "near miss," no matter how minor, must be reported to the site/unit supervisor immediately for appropriate action. The supervisor is responsible for taking appropriate follow-up action, including contacting the emergency response coordinator and getting medical attention for the injured. For minor and medium risk incidents, the supervisor is also responsible for completing an investigation report and recommending appropriate corrective actions. The report shall be reviewed and approved by department manager before implementation of corrective actions. For high risk incidents, the investigation shall be led by the department manager. Members of the investigation team shall include the site/unit supervisor and other members as required.*

The primary purpose of the accident investigation is to identify the cause(s) of the accident, incident or "near miss" and take action to prevent a similar occurrence in the future. It should be a fact-finding and not a fault-finding exercise. Hence it should focus on what failed to function well and not who failed to do what.

Near-misses should also be investigated as if they actually happened. A near-miss is an unplanned event that did not result in harm to people or damage to property and environment but had the potential to do so (if not for luck).

There are many tools used in incidents investigation in order to get to the appropriate root cause. Without getting to the root cause of an incident and correcting it, the incident is certain to repeat and probably with greater consequence.

One of these tools, called '5 Whys', is simple but effective.'5 Whys' relies on an investigation team analyzing a problem to come to the conclusion as to what the root causes are. In doing this, technical experts in the process that was disturbed should be present and help to drill down through the symptoms to get to the root cause. The '5 Whys' work by asking 'why' something happened, getting the answer and then asking 'why' again and again, until you come up with the real root cause of the problem.

There are several more advanced and sophisticated tools for incident investigation, such as tripod-beta, tap-root, root-cause tree etc. These have patented computer soft wares and you need some days of training to be able to start using them.

2.6 Hazardous Materials

Hazardous materials are those that could cause harm to people or damage to the environment. They do these either by:

- Being corrosive, visibly destroying body tissue on contact or;
- Poisoning when ingested or;
- Displacing the air to be inhaled or;
- Explosion, forceful impact.

There are many types of hazardous materials and they include the following:

- Carcinogens – chemical or physical agents that cause cancer;
- Corrosive materials – cause visible destruction of body tissues;
- Toxic materials –may damage organs such as liver, nervous system or blood;
- Irritants – cause reversible inflammatory effects on body tissue at the site of contact;
- Flammable materials – have the potential to readily ignite and burn in air;

- Explosive materials – decompose under conditions of mechanical shock, elevated temperature or chemical action, resulting in the release of large volumes of gases.

Obtaining information on hazardous materials – There are four common sources of information on hazardous materials:

1. Material Safety Data Sheets (MSDSs): MSDSs contain information on physical data, health and fire hazards, spill procedures, handling procedures and first aid requirements. Manufacturers of materials are by law required to provide MSDS on sale or delivery.
2. Container labels also provide a great deal of safety information on the contents.
3. Chemical catalogs from suppliers often contain useful safety information.
4. Internet offers a great deal of information.

Using Material Safety Data Sheets – MSDS should contain the following information:

Identity

- Name of the material
- Name, address and phone numbers of the supplier
- Chemical formula

Physical Characteristics

- Boiling point – low boiling flammable liquids present special fire hazards
- Vapor pressure – high values mean easy inhalation
- Vapor density – high density means vapors accumulate in low areas
- Water solubility
- Appearance and odor
- Specific gravity
- Water reactivity – important for cleanup operations

Special Hazards

- Flashpoint –lowest temperature at which it can vaporize to form an ignitable mixture with air
- Auto-ignition temperature – lowest temperature at which material will ignite spontaneously
- Fire-fighting information – which extinguishing material to use (foam, carbon dioxide, dry chemical)
- Explosive limits – maximum concentrations of vapors allowed

Reactivity Data

- Stability and reaction paths of dangerous decomposition
- Health hazard data
- Exposure route – absorption, inhalation etc

Health symptoms – carcinogen, irritant, corrosive etc

First aid requirements

Personal Protective Equipment& Hygiene

- Eye protection, hand protection, body protection etc
- Ventilation requirement
- Hygiene procedure – washing hands after contact etc

Waste Material Disposal

- Protective equipment to use
- Spill clean-up requirement
- Disposal method

Safe Handling of Hazardous Materials–The following are the requirements for safe handling of hazardous materials:

- No hazardous materials should be taken delivery of without the appropriate material safety data sheet (MSDS). The MSDS should be conspicuously displayed where the materials are stored.

- Accurate inventory of materials in stock should be available and readily updated. This will help workers to have information on the risk they are exposed to. In addition, this inventory will help in planning required emergency response resources.
- All materials should be clearly labeled. Original manufacturer's label must not be removed or defaced. Hazardous materials not in the original manufactures'containers must be labeled.
- Materials must always be stored and segregated in line with the requirements of the MSDS.
- Personal protective equipment (PPE) must be used as specified in the MSDS.
- Exhaust ventilation, fans, blowers and proper handling procedures shall be used to keep personnel from breathing hazardous vapors and/or dust. Respiratory protection shall be provided and used when necessary.
- Fire extinguishers shall be available.
- Eye wash stations must be installed in the vicinity where hazardous materials are stored and used.

2.7 Material Handling

The general safety rules and requirements regarding material handling are as follows:

Lifting by Hand (manual handling) – As much as possible, manual material handling should be discouraged. If unavoidable, the size, shape, weight and disposition of materials to be lifted should first be assessed. Before commencement of lifting, the proper personal protective equipment (PPE) should be worn.

There are six steps to safe lifting:

1. Place feet apart– comfortably spread to give greater stability
2. Keep back straight, nearly vertical-bending the knees
3. Firmly grip the material, using the full palm (as fingers alone have very little power) and keeping it close to the body
4. Lift the load smoothly, first to knee level, then waist level

5. Move forward, without twisting, keeping the load close to the waist and keeping head up (without looking at the load). If there is need to turn, turn by moving the feet (never twisting)
6. Set the load down by first at waist level or knee level and then floor.

When two or more people carry a material, they should adjust it so that the load rides level. When long sections of material (e.g. pipe) are carried, the load should be carried on the same shoulder and all the people should walk in step. One person should be designated to give the signal when to lift and drop.

For cylindrical materials like drums and barrels, it is recommended that a hand truck or other type of material handling equipment be used. If it is necessary to roll a drum or barrel, it should be pushed against the sides with both hands. To change directions, the drum or barrel should be stopped, the direction changed by grabbing the upper and lower rim seams and movement re-started. When uplifting the drum, the above six safe lifting steps should be followed.

For long objects like pipes, it is important that obstructions to be encountered be determined before lifting is started. If there are overhead obstructions, the object should be carried at the same level with the front end low so it does not catch the objects. If it is to be carried on shoulders, the front end should be held as high as possible to avoid striking other employees, especially when going around corners.

Compressed gas cylinders should be transported on a hand or motorized truck, suitably secured to keep them from falling. For very short distances they may be rolled on the bottom edge.

Lifting by Hand Trucks – In general, hand trucks should be kept under control at all times. They should be used at safe speed (no running), avoiding horseplay, and no riders allowed on them. Loads should be packed securely, avoiding overhanging. Aisles and loading areas should always be kept clear and after use, trucks should be stored in designated areas (not in aisles).Materials should not be loaded as to obstruct clear view of the person pushing the truck. And it is important not to pull (but push).

For one axle hand trucks, heavy materials should be placed below higher ones in order to keep the center of gravity of the load as low as possible.

For two axle trucks, the materials should be loaded evenly to prevent tipping and arranged so they will not fall if accidently bumped.

Use of Forklift - Only trained and authorized operators shall be permitted to operate forklifts. Training should include lecture, instructor led field demonstration and workplace evaluation.

Forklifts should be inspected annually by a competent person and be inspected by the operator before each use (or at least daily).

Hazardous moving parts such as chains, sprocket drives and gears shall be guarded to protect the operator in his normal operating position. Exposed tires should have guards that will stop particles from being thrown at the operator. All forklifts should have roll-over protection. Relieve valve shall be installed for all hydraulically-driven lifting systems and suitable stops provided to prevent travel over of the carriage.

Forklifts should be equipped with seat belts and ABC fire extinguishers.

Forklifts should never be loaded above their rated capacities and the loads should not be stacked as to block the operators view.

Forklifts should be equipped with horns and back-up alarms. Diesel or gasoline engine-driven forklifts should be used in adequately ventilated areas only.

Personnel should not be allowed under elevated loads. Forklifts shall not be left unattended while running or the fork is in the up position.

Forklifts should not be used for any purpose other than what they are designed to do (e.g. using the forks as hoist). And when ascending or descending grades in excess of 10%, loaded forklifts shall be driven with the load tilted backwards.

2.8 Extreme Temperatures Stress

Extreme temperature stress can either be heat stress or cold stress.

Heat Stress occurs when the body cannot cool itself enough to maintain a healthy temperature. Workers who are exposed to extreme heat (for example in fire fighting) or work in hot environments (like the desert in summer) may be at risk of heat stress. Heat stress can result into heat stroke, heat exhaustion, heat cramps or heat rashes.

Heat stroke starts when the body becomes unable to control its temperature, it rises above 40.5 degree C and the body's vital systems begin to shut down. The victim may appear confused, lose balance, collapse and lose consciousness. If this happens, the temperature should be reduced rapidly in order to prevent permanent disability or fatality.

Heat exhaustion occurs when there is excessive sweating which may reduce the blood volume. If care is not taken it may result into heat stroke. Common symptoms of heat exhaustion are paleness and sweating, rapid heart rate, muscle cramps (in the abdomen and limbs), headache, nausea, vomiting, dizziness or fainting.

Heat cramps occurs when the body gets depleted of salt and water. Common symptoms include muscle pains or spasms (in the abdomen and limbs).

Heat rash is a skin irritation caused by excessive sweating, often referred to as prickly heat.

Heat stress can be prevented by scheduling work in high temperature areas for cooler months of the year or cooler hours of the day. If the work must be carried out during high temperature periods the following precautions should be taken;

- Body protection should be light-colored, loose-fitting, breathable clothing such as cotton (rather than non-breathing synthetic clothing).
- Frequent rest-break periods should be taken, with break areas being shaded and well ventilated.
- Workers should be encouraged to drink water frequently, even when not thirsty (avoiding alcoholic drinks).
- New employees who have not worked in hot temperature environments should be deliberately acclimatized. They should be exposed to about 25% of normal exposure on the first day and gradually adjusted upwards over a period of say 5 days.
- Buddy system should be employed and hence no worker should be allowed to work alone. Workers should be monitoring each other for early signs of heat stress.
- Appropriate training should be provided to personnel on prevention, recognizing early symptoms, the needed first aid and how to get emergency medical care.

If heat cramp is noticed, the victim should stop work activity, sit quietly in a cool place, increase fluid intake and rest a few hours before returning to work (if condition improves).

If heat exhaustion has already set in, the victim should be taken to a cool area and made to lie down. The outer clothing should be removed and skin wet with cool water or wet cloths. If he or she is conscious, fluid intake should be increased while medical assistance is sought.

In a situation where the victim has already got a heat stroke, an ambulance should be called immediately. While waiting for the ambulance, he or she should be taken to a shaded, well ventilated area, clothes removed, body wetted while fanning continuously.

Workers on the other hand that are exposed to extreme cold or work in cold environments may be at risk of cold stress. When temperatures drop below normal, wind speed increases, and heat rapidly leaves the body, this may lead to serious adverse health problems. Cold stress can result into hypothermia, frost bite, trench foot and chilblains.

Hypothermia occurs when the body starts to lose heat faster than it can produce. Prolonged exposure to cold will eventually use up the body's stored energy. When the body temperature gets too low it may affect the brain and the victim may not be able to think or move well. Common early symptoms are shivering, fatigue, loss of coordination, confusion and disorientation. Common late symptoms are stoppage of shivering, blue skin, dilated pupils, slow pulse, slow breathing and loss of consciousness.

Frostbite occurs when a body part is frozen. The parts of the body most commonly affected are the fingers, toes, nose, ears, cheeks, and chin. It causes a loss of feeling in the affected areas and can permanently damage body tissues, and in severe cases may result to amputation. Common symptoms are numbness, tingling, aching, paleness or skin coloring, and waxy skin.

Trench foot occurs when the foot is exposed to wet and cold conditions for prolonged period. And sometimes it can occur at temperatures as high as 60 degrees F if the feet are constantly wet and hence lose heat 25-times faster than dry feet. When this happens, the body goes into defensive mode. It tries to prevent heat loss, and constricts blood vessels to shut down circulation in the feet. This causes the skin tissue to begin to die because of lack of oxygen and nutrients and due to the buildup of toxic products. Common symptoms of trench foot are skin reddening, numbness, cramps, swelling, tingling pain, blisters or ulcers, hemorrhage under the skin, and gangrene.

Chilblains occur by the repeated exposure of skin to temperatures just above freezing to as high as 60 degrees F. The cold exposure damages the capillary beds in the skin. Common symptoms of chilblains are redness, itching, blistering, inflammation, and ulceration.

Cold stress can be prevented by scheduling work in cold temperature areas for warmer months of the year or warmer hours of the day. If the work must be carried out during cold temperature periods the following precautions should be taken;

- Body protection should be appropriate warm clothing (several layers as needed) protecting the ears, face, hands and feet in extremely cold weather.
- Amount of time workers are exposed to the cold weather should be limited and warm locations should be provided for break periods.
- Extra workers should be assigned for long, demanding jobs in the cold.
- Warm drinks should be provided for workers.
- Workers at risk should be closely monitored.
- Buddy system should be employed and hence no worker should be allowed to work alone. Workers should be monitoring each other for early signs of cold stress.
- Appropriate training should be provided to personnel on worker risk, prevention, recognizing early symptoms, and treatment.

If a worker gets hypothermia, he/she should be moved to a warm shelter, every wet clothing removed and medical care requested without delay. The body of the victim should then be warmed in the order, chest, neck, head and groin using electric blanket (if available) or use skin-to-skin contact under loose, dry layers of blankets, clothing, towels or sheets. If victim is conscious, warm beverages may help increase the body temperature (but alcoholic beverages are prohibited). In a situation where the victim has no pulse, cardiopulmonary resuscitation (CPR) should be started.

If a worker gets frostbite, the victim should be moved into a warm room as soon as possible. The victim should not be allowed to walk on frostbitten feet or toes as this will likely increase the damage. The affected part should also be warmed either by immersion in warm water (take note, not hot water) or using body heat. The affected part should not be massaged to avoid damaging the external tissues.

Workers suffering from trench foot should remove shoes/boots and wet socks, dry their feet and avoid walking on the feet, as this may cause tissue damage. For chilblains, the victim should avoid scratching; slowly warm the skin and use corticosteroid creams to relieve itching and swelling. If blisters and ulcers occur, they should be kept clean and covered, while being treated.

2.9 Fire Prevention

For a fire to start, three conditions must be met at the same time: fuel, oxygen (or oxidizer) and ignition source. Fire prevention consists of making sure that all these three elements do not exist at the same time.

A fuel is any material that burns. The higher the temperature, the easier and quicker they burn. Common fuels in the petroleum industry are liquid and gaseous hydrocarbons, alcohols, wood, paper, and chemicals of all sorts.

Oxygen is commonly available in the atmosphere. Oxidizers are substances capable of releasing oxygen to a fire. Common oxidizers include: acids, especially nitric and chloric acids; chlorine dioxide; potassium permanganate and potassium chlorate.

An ignition source can be: a spark; static electricity; arcs from electrical equipment, faulty or otherwise; a lit cigarette; open flame; welding arc; hot light bulbs etc.

Recent studies indicate that the spread or propagation of a fire is also dependent on a fourth factor – the chemical chain reactions that can occur as a result of heat produced by the fire. A fire will not always start when the three elements meet, unless all three are present in the required proportions. For example, vapors from a flammable liquid must be mixed with a certain amount of air in order to ignite and propagate a flame.

The lowest concentration at which a fuel/air mixture will burn is called lower flammable limit. Below this there is too little fuel (the mixture is too lean) to burn. On the other hand, the upper flammable limit is the highest concentration at which a fuel/air mixture will burn. Above this there is not enough oxygen (the mixture is too rich) to support burning.

There is also a temperature below which sufficient vapors from a liquid can form an ignitable mixture with air. This is called the flash point for that liquid. All liquids with flash point below 100 degrees F are classified as flammables and those above 100 degrees F are combustibles.

Storage & Handling - Since it is impossible to eliminate oxygen from the atmosphere, fire prevention should start from safe storage and handling of materials. Information from the material safety data sheet (MSDS) and container labelling should give the fire risk, the storage and handling requirements.

Sources of ignition should be eliminated where flammable and combustible materials are being handled or stored. Adequate clearance should be maintained between flammable/combustible materials and electric lighting/heating units. Incompatible materials (e.g. flammables and oxidizers) shall not be kept together. As much as possible, the amount of flammables and combustibles stored or handled should be reduced to the barest minimum.

For large amounts of flammables and combustibles, the best location to store them is in a separate outside building. If this is not possible, then a suitable flammable storage cabinet or inside storage room should be built. Flammable materials should not be stored directly under the sun.

Appropriate warning signs (for example, "Flammable materials" "No open flames" "No Smoking") should be displayed where these materials are stored.

Control of Ignition Sources – Equipment and activities that have potential for ignition sources shall be prohibited around flammable or combustible materials and this includes:

- Checking that electrical equipment do not have defects that could create sparks or arcs. Temporary electrical wiring shall be carried out by competent persons.
- Smoking should be permitted only in designated areas.
- Effective grounding should be done when carrying out activities where static electricity could be an ignition source.
- Special permission should be obtained before carrying out activities or operations that have potentials for ignition sources. Such permission should only be given by supervisors with requisite competence, having checked and satisfied themselves that flammable/combustible materials are not and will not be present within the period the permission is granted.

Emergency Procedures and Equipment – Part of fire prevention is to stop the propagation of fire when it starts. To do this, clear and concise procedure on what personnel should do on noticing fire/smoke should be posted in conspicuous locations in the work site/facility. This procedure should include telephone numbers of the closest fire stations.

Emergency exit routes and directions to safe areas should be clearly marked, well lit and should be connected to an emergency electricity lighting source.

In addition, appropriate fire extinguishers should be placed in strategic locations and personnel trained on how to use them. The following are types of fire extinguishers (for different types of materials on fire);

- Class A type – water-based fire extinguisher, used for common solids (like wood and paper).
- Class ABC multipurpose dry chemical – displaces oxygen and smothers the flame.
- Class ABC halon 1211 – inhibits chain reactions of a fire.
- Class BC – carbon dioxide displaces air and cuts off the oxygen supply.

2.10 Journey Management

In the petroleum industry, there is enormous risk associated with the transportation of workers, equipment and materials. To minimize this risk in every journey an organization should have a journey management process, the objectives of which should include:

- Challenge the business need for every journey made;
- Limit personnel exposure by ensuring that only essential journeys are made and combining journeys where feasible;
- Select the most appropriate mode of journey in every circumstance;
- Ensure that only competent and fit-for-work drivers operate company or contractor vehicles;
- Effective monitoring of active journeys;
- Emergency response (in case of incidents, vehicle breakdowns, overdue arrivals).

Responsibilities – A journey management process should appoint and train relevant personnel for the following roles in journey management:

- Journey Managers - these are the personnel who are responsible for leading the journeys (this could either be the driver or the most senior personnel in a trip). His or her responsibilities include: justifying the need for a journey; preparing a journey plan and getting it approved;

ensuring that control measures are in place for identified risks of the journey; ensuring that the requirements of the journey are adhered to; and if deviations arise while executing the journey, conduct a risk assessment and ensure control measures are in place.

- Journey Coordinators – these are permanent positions and should be personnel who manage the organization's fleet of transport vehicles. His responsibility include: controlling all journeys; issuing the approved journey plan to the journey manager; ensuring that the journey vehicle is fit, and has adequate emergency response resources, including functional means of communication; conducting briefing for the driver prior to departure, explaining the identified risks and agreed control measures; ensuring that drivers are competent and fit; dispatching the vehicle, monitoring its movement until journey is completed and logged-in; and in case of emergency, contacting the emergency response coordinator.

- Journey Authorizers – these are operational managers or superintendents of facilities or work sites. Their responsibilities include: challenging the need for every journey, and approving or rejecting; instructing on alternatives for journey plans presented for approval; approving journeys being undertaken at odd hours or in adverse weathers; approving any deviations to original journey plans.

- Drivers (if they are not the journey managers).

- Emergency Response Coordinators – these do not need to be permanent positions. They can be in rotation by senior company personnel to provide 24 hours coverage to activate emergency response when notified that workers on journey have encountered problems ranging from vehicle breakdown to accidents.

Journey Assessment and Preparation – The process should also specify mode of assessment and preparation of journeys. Before any journey is embarked on it should be challenged to determine its operational/business need and risks associated with the proposed mode of travel. If the purpose of the journey can be accomplished by alternative means it should be cancelled. On the other hand, if the journey must be undertaken, the modes of transport shall be considered in the order: train, air, company bus, operational vehicle.

If operational vehicle is chosen as the best means of accomplishing the journey, the route should be planned, putting into consideration the inherent hazards like road condition, accident records, third party drivers' behavior, traffic congestion, time of travel (day or night), weather conditions, security etc. For all identified hazards, control measures should be put in place, and documented. The condition of the vehicle and driver to be used should also be assessed using approved checklists. All these should be part of the journey plan that should be approved by the authorizer.

Journey Execution – The journey coordinators should discuss the details of the journey plan with the journey manager and the driver via a tool box meeting. The toolbox meetings attendees will sign to indicate understanding and a copy of the journey plan should be handed over to the journey manager. During the toolbox meeting the following should also be agreed; method of monitoring progress of the journey, emergency response notification and rest intervals/locations. While the journey is being executed and there is need to deviate from the approved plan, the journey manager should get approval from the authorizer. At the end of the journey lessons learnt should be documented and possibly communicated to other personnel.

Additional Road Transport Safety – Road transportation is the single leading cause of fatalities in the petroleum industry. To minimize this:

- Vehicles used should be fit for purpose and well maintained. The maintenance routine as instructed by the manufacturer should be adhered to as a minimum. The vehicle should be inspected regularly by the user with an approved checklist, and defects corrected promptly. In addition, before the commencement of any journey the driver should check that all safety equipment (including the spare tire) is in place and that all lights are functional.
- Vehicles used in exploration activities and in rough terrain shall be four wheel drives and in addition, have rollover protection.
- All personnel who drive company vehicles should, in addition to possession of driver's license, undergo defensive driving training that is tailored to the peculiar operation environment.

- Drivers should comply with all applicable rules, and traffic signs (including speed limits).
- Driving under the influence of alcohol or drugs, and use of cell phone while on the wheel should be prohibited.
- Driver and all passengers must use their seat belts at all times while on a journey.

HelicopterTransport Safety – Personnel who travel with a helicopter should in general follow the instructions of the pilot and never pressure him to do anything against his judgment. In addition:

- Passengers should have valid helicopter underwater escape training (HUET) or similar certification.
- Prior to boarding the aircraft, all passengers should undergo safety briefing and this should be specific to the type of craft being used.
- Ear defenders and life vests should be worn before boarding the helicopter and throughout the duration of the flight.
- Personnel should keep clear of the landing pad until the helicopter has landed and the pilot signals that people can approach.
- Extreme caution should be exercised when approaching or leaving a helicopter to avoid being harmed by the rotor. As a general rule, follow the direction of the pilot or approach from the front or side of the aircraft in full view of the pilot. Never approach from the back. The rotors are generally about 2.5 meters above grade, but this clearance could be shortened in uneven grounds or in windy weather due to the flexibility of the rotor. Hence, if the ground is uneven, passengers should approach/depart from downhill locations and in full view of the pilot. In windy weather, it is advisable to stoop while approaching or departing.
- Dangerous goods (which shall be specified during pre-boarding safety briefing) shall not be carried in helicopters. Approved baggage should be weighed and transported in the aircraft baggage compartment (and never in the passenger cabin).
- Keep firm grip on objects being carried to the helicopter and remove hats to avoid being blown away by the wave generated by the rotor.
- Long objects should be carried horizontally and below the waist.

- The total weight of passengers and baggage to be transported should be communicated to the pilot. Helicopters shall never be overloaded.
- The weighing scale used in helicopter baggage operations should be regularly calibrated in order to ensure that it weighs accurately.
- Smoking should be prohibited around or inside the helicopter.
- Once inside the aircraft, all passengers should fasten their seat belts.
- Passengers should never throw objects from the helicopter except with the permission of the pilot.

Boat Transport Safety – Accidents do occur while embarking, travelling or disembarking from boats and could often be fatal. To minimize or completely eliminate these, the boat captain or operator shall be empowered to be responsible for safety of people and goods. In addition:

- Boats that are used in the petroleum industry shall have been properly surveyed and have valid license in line with the law of the country where it is being operated.
- Boat captain or operator shall have a valid operational license for the capacity and type of craft operated.
- Regular inspection should be conducted to ensure that marine safety equipment are available and operational and these include:
    o Personal flotation devices (the number of life jackets on board shall at least be equal to the number of crew and passengers allowed to be carried by the operational license. There should also be lifebuoys with lines.);
    o Telecommunication equipment;
    o Flares and other devices on a vessel that can be used to attract attention;
    o Position identification systems installed on a vessel;
    o Anchors and other devices carried on a vessel that may be used to maintain the vessel's position or stability;
    o Paddles and other alternative means of propulsion in case of engine breakdown;
    o Fire extinguishers and sand buckets;
    o Navigation lights;
    o Horn.

- Boat captain or operator shall have a valid operational license for the capacity and type of craft operated.
- Prior to the start of every journey, passengers should undergo safety orientation specific to the type of craft being used.
- Personal floatation devices (PFD) should be worn during embarkation/disembarkation and throughout the duration of the journey.
- Safe access should be used for embarking or disembarking from a boat. Personnel should never be allowed to jump in or out.
- Passengers should not embark or disembark from a boat unless the captain or operator has given signal for them to do so.
- In the unlikely event of someone falling into the water, the first person witnessing that should shout 'man over board' and a lifebuoy with line should be thrown to the victim (this should be part of the organization emergency response procedures).
- Smoking shall not be permitted while on board a boat

Chapter 3

EXPLORATION OPERATIONS

3.1 Health, Allergies and First Aid

There are few activities that expose workers to a wide variety of hazards as much as exploration operations. And these take place in remote locations with limited access to established medical care. It is therefore important at the planning stage to anticipate possible problems and put in place effective solutions to workers health and allergy problems that might arise.

Potential employees should pass medical examination prior to employment, specifying that they are fit for work in such challenging locations. Some type of confidential health forms for all crews should be completed and kept with the exploration party chiefs. For each employee, this form should list ailments, allergies, adverse reactions to medicines (e.g. chloroquine), medication required, size and frequency of dosages, circumstances that may cause onset of symptoms, recent surgeries or injuries, special dietary requirements and if anything requires special physician attention (and possibly name and contact details of personal physicians).All personnel in the field should keep their tetanus inoculations up to date. These measures have to be taken because it may not be sufficient to rely upon personnel to take suitable precautions to sustain their health while out there in remote locations. Such things as allergic reactions, if not handled timely or even prevented can result in seizures, comas and even death. In some circumstances, co-workers should be alerted to watch for adverse reactions and should know what remedial actions to take.

Extra precautions should be taken with clean drinking water, environmental cleanliness, and personal hygiene as infectious diseases can disrupt work activities when they set in. Wastes should be collected and disposed of properly.

There should be well-stocked first aid boxes and wilderness first aid book. It is recommended that every exploration crew with ten or more personnel and a distance of 20 minutes or more from a hospital should have a certified nurse and a means of evacuating injured persons to a hospital. The contact details of the hospital being used by the organization should be prominently displayed at the site. In addition, every employee should have valid first aid and CPR certificates. All minor injuries should be treated promptly so that they do not develop into major problems. Personnel whose jobs have potential for severe wounds should always carry pressure bandages while in the field.

For extreme temperature stress, refer to section 2.8.

3.2 Camp Management

Safety in the management of camp is a matter of common sense combined with adequate preparation. It is important that camp bosses be safety conscious, proactively recognize and prevent hazards.

Location and Layout – Before determining the location of an exploration camp, it is important to look for information on the proposed site (either by talking to people who have worked there before or through internet searches). Ask questions with regards to security, climate, wild animals, insects' infestations, relevant laws/regulations, and hospitability of neighboring population.

Camps should be constructed: in safe locations removed from environmental threats such as flood, avalanches, sand storms, falling trees, animal trails; to have minimum environmental impact; with fire breaks of at least 6 meters between structures and between outer structures and wild vegetation.

An emergency tent/structure should be located far enough so that in case the camp is destroyed it should be safe enough. This tent should have at least three days of emergency ration (depending on how far the camp is from the organization's base or nearest re-supply point).

Camp structures should be located in a straight line (and not in a circle) so that if a wild animal is to be shot there would be nobody in the line of fire while inside the tents. They should be in line with the prevailing wind direction and not diagonal. The layout should take into consideration vulnerability to flooding, forest fires, avalanches, rock falls, sand storms, falling trees, and wild animal trails.

Flammable materials (including fuel dump) should be located down or cross of prevailing wind directions away from the living structures with effective fire break. The kitchen structure should be about fifty meters away from the sleeping area and same distance from the flammable materials storage.

Garbage should be disposed and burnt at least 100 meters away (downwind of the fuel dump) so that bears and wild animals looking for leftovers will not stray into the sleeping tents.

If electrical supply to the camp is by generator, it should be located down wind. It is preferable to use diesel-powered generators rather than gasoline-powered in order to minimize the risk of fire. Power lines should be buried at a safe depth (with route marked) or suspended from insulated poles at a safe height and protected from damage by vehicles. All wiring should be done by a licensed electrician and should be inspected regularly. In addition, all outlets should be installed with over-current protection (or ground fault circuit interruption) and all electronic equipment protected by surge protectors.

Fire Hazards–For a fire to start and burn, it must have fuel, oxygen and ignition source. The best way to prevent a fire is to remove any of these three components. The following precautions should be taken to reduce the risk of fire in a camp:

- Arrange the camp (as in location and layout, above).
- Follow precautions in section 2.9 (fire prevention).

Fires are classed as:
A: Fires in ordinary solid materials (e.g. paper, wood, dry vegetation)
B: Fires in liquids (e.g. petroleum products)
C: Fires in electrical equipment
D: Fires in combustible metals (e.g. sodium, magnesium).

A, B, or C fires are the most likely to happen in a camp, hence dry chemical powders (commonly called ABC fire extinguishers) should be readily available. One extinguisher should be located in each structure, in visible locations and free from obstruction. Each structure should also be equipped with a smoke detector and carbon monoxide monitor. Heat detectors should be located in the kitchen. All these extinguishers, detectors and monitors should be inspected regularly.

Fire Arms – Fire arms could be required because of wild animals. But this should be acquired and kept in line with the law. If the law allows it, firearms and ammunition should be stored in a secure, safe place in the camp under the supervision of a responsible and/or certified person. The organization should have firearm safety systems and only trained/authorized individuals should be allowed to use firearms.

As a general rule, loaded firearms should never be transported in any vehicle (including boats and aircrafts). The chamber should be kept empty and the ammunition stored in a separate place. In some countries, the laws requires that all the ammunitions be kept in the custody of the driver (or captain/ pilot) of the transport vehicle (or boat/aircraft) while the empty weapon is kept in the baggage compartment. It is also important to adequately protect the weapon while being transported to avoid damage to sights and the alignment. While in the field the gun can be hand-carried in a back pack but the weapon separated from the ammunition.

In the camp, the firearm and matching ammunition could be kept in the same container but under lock and key. If the camp is unattended, and the firearm is to be left behind, it is advisable to keep the weapon in a nearby (but secure) location so as not to get back and find a wild animal and the gun in the same location.

When there is the need to fire the gun in the camp it should be aimed such that there is no tent where people could be is in the line of fire. It is advisable to give the animal every opportunity to go away and firing should be the last resort if the live of personnel are threatened.

Horse playing or pointing the gun at personnel should be prohibited and contravention should attract a consequence of being sent out of the camp.

Sanitation and Hygiene – Sanitation facilities should comply with applicable laws, as a minimum. Small, short term camps should employ mobile toilets and efficient means of waste disposal. Larger and longer-term camps should have a septic tank and possibly small-sized sewage treatment plants.

Drugs, Alcohol and Tobacco –There should be a policy declaring zero tolerance to possession and use of hard drugs or the abuse of prescription drugs in camp. Users must be removed immediately without warning.

Alcohol policy should vary from nation to nation and company to company, from outright ban to use outside work hours. However, there should zero tolerance to alcohol abuse. Medical personnel should refrain completely from use of alcohol.

Smoking policy should designate smoking areas and metal containers for disposal of cigarette stubs. It should never be allowed in sleeping quarters and cigarette stubs must not be disposed of except in designated containers (to avoid starting bush fires).

These policies should be signed by company chief executives, communicated to every employee during the orientation and strictly enforced.

Wild Animals, Insects and Diseases Control – Wild animals and insects have the potential to make a camp uncomfortable, unsafe and unhealthy. Structures should be constructed such that animals and reptiles do not have loopholes through which they gain access. Insect screens should be installed in all shutters.

Cleanliness and waste disposal minimizes insects' invasion. The same applies to wild animals (like bears). When animals discover and feed somewhere, they will keep coming back. Ensure that garbage is well contained and incinerated effectively. Regular fumigation should be carried out as it is an additional defense against wild animals, reptiles and insects.

Workers should be trained not to feed or attract wild animals or bring them into the camp. And when the animals appear in the camp, they should not be alarmed or provoked. As a last resort, firearms should be used to kill wild animals when they become aggressive and threaten the lives of workers.

Communications – A camp should have two reliable means of communication (the primary and a back-up), like GSM phone, two-way radio, satellite phone. The communication means should be tested on a daily basis by at least using them to make contact with the base office. Every personnel should be trained on the use of the communication equipment and know their locations.

There should also be means of communication (the primary and a back-up) between the field crews and the camp and between the different the crews themselves.

Medical Equipment – Every camp should have a well stocked medical treatment kit, a certified nurse (if the distance to the closest hospital is more than 20 minutes drive), a vehicle for evacuating injured or sick person, and contact details of the company clinic/doctor conspicuously displayed. The location of the medical kit should be known to every personnel. In addition, every employee should be in possession of valid first aid and CPR certificates.

3.3 Hand and Powered Tools

There are several hand and powered tools that could be put into use during exploration operations depending on the activity being performed. Before using any of these, workers should be familiar with the safe operating requirements. They should be provided with adequate instructions on the function of the tool, possible dangers, correct operating procedure and required PPEs (see section 2.3).

Axes and Knives – Axes should have blade protectors or sheath while being transported. When carrying an unprotected axe, hold handle immediately below the head with the blade facing outward for maximum protection in the event of a fall. It is safer to choose a long-handled axe and ensure it is sharp. The long handle allows the axe to hit the ground and not the carrier's leg. A sharp axe will reduce the energy required and hence also reduce accidents attributable to fatigue. The axe head and handle should be checked to ensure that they tight fit before each use. It is advisable to soak the axe head area in water overnight and insert a new wedge that fits tightly. The work area should also be inspected and cleared of obstructions before cutting commences. While working, both hands should be used to grip the handle firmly while maintaining good footing. Other workers should maintain a good distance away from the cutting activity in case the axe head flies off.

Chainsaws – Chainsaws are used for felling trees and cutting woods. Very serious accidents do result if they are not used properly. Chainsaw accidents are commonly caused by contact with the blade while it is running. As with any other equipment, it can be used safely, effectively and efficiently if some basic rules are followed. Some of the rules are as follows;

- Workers should use chain saws that they have been trained to use properly and safely.
- Before use, the owner's manual should be read carefully and understood.
- Chainsaws should be operated, adjusted and maintained according to the manufacturer's directions.
- Prior to each use (at least once daily), the following should be checked:
  o The chain guard removed and the machine inspected for loose, damaged, worn, missing parts, and leaks;
  o Chain tension and the guide bar for tightness;
  o Spark arrestor in the muffler (to reduce the risk of fire);
  o Chain, for proper lubrication;
  o Chain catcher is in place (to reduce the risk of injury if chain breaks).
- The chain brake should be engaged before starting the saw.
- Chainsaws should only be operated in well ventilated areas.
- Appropriate PPEs should be worn and this includes body protection (but no loose clothing to prevent entanglement with moving parts), hard hats (possibly with chin strap), steel-toed safety shoes, hand gloves, ear defenders and safety glasses.
- Saws should be operated only when the operator is well rested to avoid fatigue related incidents.
- The surroundings – weather conditions, terrain, wildlife, buildings, vegetation, power lines, other people, vehicles and equipment – should be checked before commencement of cutting.
- The chain saw should be carried by its front handle, with the muffler away from your body and the guard bar pointing behind you so that if you trip you would not fall on the equipment.
- The weight, power and bar length should be suitable for the size of tree to be cut.
- The equipment should be held firmly with both hands and foot standing in a well-balanced position when cutting.
- The equipment should not be refueled while running.

- It should not be started when it is resting against any part of a person's body and it should not run unattended.
- People should not stand directly behind the saw to avoid injury from sudden kick-back.
- The direction the tree being cut should be checked before commencement and as the cutting progresses.
- The chainsaw should not be carried about whilst it is running.
- The muffler is hot when the equipment is running and hence to avoid burn injury should not be touched.
- No chainsaw operator should work alone.
- To ensure the operator and others are not injured by the falling tree, it is important the lean of the tree is accurately judged, and a retreat route is planned. The ground surrounding the tree and along the escape route should be cleared and the cutter should always look out for falling debris. In addition, special care should be taken to make a proper undercut and leave an adequate hinge of wood to maintain control of falling direction. And most importantly, no one should be in the immediate area where the cutting is taking place (aside the operator of the chainsaw) and everyone in the vicinity should be made aware of the activity.

Geophysical Equipment – Workers should take particular care when working with geophysical equipment as conductor wires used in induced polarization surveys become energized during use and may cause fatalities. When surveys are in process warning signs should be posted in road crossings, particularly in inhabited places.

Electrical Equipment – Electrically powered tools should only be maintained by competent people. Ground fault circuit interrupters should be used for portable electrical equipment, temporary wiring and in wet areas. Equipment should be inspected for damage before each use. Defective ones should be put away and labeled and should never be brought back to service until repaired.

3.4 Handling, Transportation and Use of Explosives

The handling, transportation, use and disposal of explosives are governed by laws of the country in which the operation is being carried out. However, in most countries it is required that all handlers and users of explosives have "Approved Handlers" or "Shot-firer" certification.

Storage – Explosives should be securely stored under lock and key. The conditions for storage of various quantities are specified in the laws of the respective countries. These laws should also prescribe construction materials for the magazines and methods to secure explosives against theft. While in storage, explosives and detonators must be segregated.

Approved handlers should keep accurate and updated records of magazine stocks and this should include;

- The description (including name) and quantity of each item stored in the magazine;
- Quantity of each item removed for a daily job;
- Quantity of each item returned upon completion of job;
- Running total of quantity of stocks on site.

Regular stock taking should be conducted to confirm that no explosive has been lost or stolen.

Transportation–Transportation of explosives has some legal requirements. In some countries the law requires notification to the government of the intended route, times and quantities to be transported on public roads. The transportation procedure should include the following:

- That it is under the control of an approved handler and well secured;
- That the vehicle is in good mechanical condition, fully enclosed, locked, fire resistant and has warning signs (diamond placards for explosives) at the front and back;
- That it is not exposed to impact, pressure shock, heat or sparks and no smoking in or around the vehicle;
- Non-essential personnel are not transported in the same vehicle;

- Adequate and correct types (ABC type) of fire extinguishers are carried in the explosives vehicle;
- Detonators and explosives are not carried in the same vehicle unless they are effectively separated;
- Vehicles are never left unattended, never loaded beyond their capacity and only the quantity of explosives needed is moved;
- Loaded explosives vehicle is never subjected to maintenance or repair;
- The vehicle driver should be licensed for transportation of hazardous substances.

Use of Explosives –

- An approved handler should be fully responsible for the conduct of blasting operations with the use of explosives. His responsibility covers all personnel and equipment in the blasting area. He must establish a "Controlled Zone" (CZ). Within a CZ the adverse effects of explosives usage are reduced or eliminated and beyond the zone, members of the public are provided with reasonable protection from the adverse effects. If there is more than one approved handler, the manager in charge should designate one of them with authorityfor the safe conduct of the blasting operation and all others must support him/her in the exercise of this authority.
- No work should be done within a blasting area (which is no less than 15 meters radius from the nearest assembled charges) without prior approval of the designated approved handler.
- During priming, placing and connection of charges only essential personnel should be in the blasting area. Strict access control and appropriate signage should be used to restrict entry of unauthorized personnel.
- Before starting charging operations, it is important to establish a safe, accessible position to place all explosives items that will be required as charging progresses. The position must be dry, away from equipment movement route and labeled. There should not be any ignition source within 15 m of holes being charged.
- Before firing a charge, the approved handler should determine that adequate protective measures have been taken for the safety of persons and protection of property and audible warning is given.

- After firing a shot, no person should re-enter the blast area until the dust, fumes and toxic gases arising from the explosion have been dispersed.
- The designated approved handler should keep adequate record of the number of shots fired, the number of misfires and the quantity/number/type of explosives used in each shot.
- In the event that any piece of explosive is found after shot-firing it should be disposed of by inserting into another blast-hole in such a manner that it is completely destroyed when the shot is fired. In same vein, a faulty detonator should be disposed of by inserting it into a primer in another blast in a manner that ensures it will be completely destroyed when the shot is fired.

3.5 Foot Travel

Before setting out on foot, it is important to ensure that all necessary equipment are in good working condition and these include:

- Suitable means of communication and a back-up (e.g. satellite/GSM phones and two-way radio);
- GPS/compass;
- Water & Food;
- Pocket knife, machete or small axe;
- Flashlight (and batteries);
- Waterproof matches and lighters;
- Extra clothing appropriate for the weather;
- Rain coats (depending on the season);
- Blanket;
- Signal flares;
- First aid kit (including necessary prescription medicines);
- Ropes;
- Personal floatation device (PFD) or life jacket if travelling in swampy locations or where there is potential of crossing shallow waters.

In addition, the following precautions should be taken:

- Check the weather forecast before setting out;

- Communicate the destination, route of travel and estimated return time to the person in charge of the site or the base radio operator;
- Mark the route of travel;
- Personnel should as much as possible travel in pairs;
- There should be a search and rescue process in place if any personnel is in danger or does not return at the estimated time.

3.6 Insects and Wild Animals

Wild Animals - Attacks by wild animals are not very common in exploration activity. However when they happen, in most instances, they are provoked because the animal:

o   Feels threatened or that its young is;

o   Is protecting food or territory;

o   Is surprised.

To minimize or eliminate the risk posed by wild animals, the above listed circumstances should be avoided. The following control measures are advised:

- Areas heavily used by wild animals or where there have been problems with wild animals in the past should be avoided;
- Personnel should be given orientation on the way to handle wild animals prevalent in their area of operation (locals, wildlife experts and internet are recommended sources of information);
- Food storage containers should conceal odors;
- Food waste should be minimized and all garbage incinerated on a daily basis;
- Use of heavily scented cosmetics should be minimized and extra caution is advised in the use and disposal menstrual pads;
- Personnel should be advised against feeding wild animals;
- Before entry into heavy bushes, it is advisable to make loud noise to alert animals of people's presence;
- People should be alert for strange smell of animals, foot prints, droppings and always look ahead for them;
- Never approach the young of animals and in the event of coming across them it is advisable to retreat in the same direction of encounter.

- When the life of personnel is at risk, fire arm could be used against an attacking animal. However, extreme caution should be exercised to ensure that people are not in the line of fire.
- In the unlikely event of being attacked or beaten by a wild animal, the victim should seek immediate medical attention to avoid infection.

Snakes–Snakes are not particularly aggressive and always strike when rattled or irritated. It is important to avoid snake bites by taking the following precautions:

- Personnel should be familiar with the various species of snakes that live in their area of operation, where and when to expect them;
- Bites are usually at the lower part of the legs and hence safety shoes should be "high-cut" leather work boots;
- The camp should be kept free of debris and clutter in order to minimize hiding place for snakes;
- Food and garbage containers should be tightly closed to avoid mouse infestation (as this attracts snakes);
- The camp should be fumigated regularly;
- Workers should be given orientation on treatment for snake bites and appropriate medicines should be part of the first aid kit stock.

Insects - Mosquitoes, flies, ticks, leeches could constitute significant nuisance in the field. To avoid being bitten by these insects:

- Personnel should use relevant repellant creams;
- Shirts and pants that cover most part of the body should be worn (if possible, these dresses should be treated with permethrin products);
- Insects screens should be installed on all doors and windows;
- Regular fumigation should be carried out in the camps;
- If working in malaria prevalent regions of the world, it is advisable to take anti malaria drugs as prescribed by a physician.

3.7 Survival

Exploration activities take place in rough and sometimes uncharted terrain. The ability to survive in such locations in extreme circumstances requires preparation and rehearsal.

- All personnel should be trained in survival techniques and possibly be supplied with a copy of survival manual.
- Each group should have a means of communication and back-up (e.g. GSM, two-way radio and satellite phone) and GPS (geographic position system).
- All vehicles should be equipped with survival kits sufficient for the number of passengers carried (same for boats and helicopters, if applicable).
- An up to date log of personnel movement should be kept at the base camp and search/rescue procedure should be in place.
- Survival kits should include:
  o Communication equipment and GPS;
  o Fire starting kit;
  o Pocket knife;
  o Compass and topographic map;
  o Notebook and pencil;
  o Dry food- nuts, raisins, dried fruits, chocolates, high energy biscuits;
  o Drinking water and fruit drinks;
  o Safety glasses;
  o Sleeping bags;
  o Reflective jackets;
  o Blanket;
  o Nylon rope;
  o First aid kit;
  o Survival manual.
- Regular drills should be held on search and rescue.

Chapter 4

DRILLING OPERATIONS

4.1 Drilling Location Preparation and Rig Move

Prior to drilling and ancillary equipment being brought in, the vegetation on the access road and the location should be cleared, the earth levelled and compacted. These are done with the use of bulldozers, graders and compactors. The conductor hole, 'rat hole' and 'mouse hole' are drilled most times with manual drilling machines. The drilling pad, the cellar pit and waste pit are then constructed. These activities are similar to those found in any other construction site and are explained in Chapter 5.

After the location is prepared, the drilling rig and ancillary equipment are loaded on trucks at the previous drill site or base yard, secured and transported to the new drilling location. Loading and unloading are lifting operations that are explained in Chapter 5.

Carrying the equipment on trucks across public highways is unusual because the loads are heavy, wide and sometimes awkward. Some of the hazards associated with this activity are:

- Vehicular accidents
- Striking fixed objects such as power poles, sign posts, trees, buildings etc.
- Overhead electrical power lines
- Unstable or slippery drill site access road.

To minimize the risks associated with rig moves, it is advisable to make use of companies specialized on such heavy lifts and transfer the risk to them. In addition:

- The route to the location should be inspected in advance for adequate vehicle access and satisfactory surface conditions.
- Local traffic authorities should be notified of the intent and the proposed route.
- Movement should as much as possible be done during low traffic periods.
- All the trucks should go in a convoy but leaving enough gaps in between, such that third party vehicles do not have to overtake the entire convoy in a stretch.
- There should be two smaller vehicles (one in the front and the other at rear of the convoy) to warn and possibly control other road users.
- Red flags should be placed at the rear end of a load (if it extends beyond the rear of the truck) and at the sides (if it is wider than the width of the truck).
- The trucks should be driven slowly and with caution.
- There should be guide men where the access is narrow and possibly use wooden poles to push up sagging overhead power lines.

4.2 Rigging Up and Location Layout

Rigging up is assembling the various components of the rig in preparation for drilling. Prior to commencement of rig-up operations, the layout of the location should be reviewed to ensure that hazards with regards to spacing and positioning of various equipment is minimized.

During the assembly of the rig, equipment and components are handled and set with forklifts and cranes. Various other activities could involve welding, flame cutting, work at height, and use of hand and power tools. Safety in each of these is explained in Chapters 5. There is however, still a challenge in managing the various work crews during separate activities simultaneously. The tool pusher or the rig foreman, having overall responsibility for safety on the rig, should control all the activities to ensure safe interface.

There should be a job safety analysis for each of the activities and work permit system (explained in Chapter 5) to ensure that each activity is properly reviewed and approved before commencement.

In addition, the following should be in place:

- Visible rig identification sign erected at entrance to site road and at all directional changes on site road (in case of emergencies, responders could easily locate the site);
- Safety signs at the gate and other prominent locations on site to indicate specific hazards (e.g. H_2S/SO_2, NO SMOKING) and PPE requirements;
- Vehicle parking location designated a minimum distance of 100 feet (30.5 m) from the well bore or a distance equal to the height of the derrick or mast (including attachments), whichever is greater;
- Windsock erected;
- Accommodation and office caravans erected in the prevailing upwind or cross wind direction of well bore;
- H_2S gas monitors, if applicable, calibrated and mounted;
- Self-contained breathing apparatus mounted at selected locations and clearly sign-posted;
- Emergency escape air packs and life lines available, if applicable;
- Escape line and anchor available;
- Escape line length twice the derrick height;
- Escape line and carrier inspected with each rig-up;
- Escape and guy wires flagged with visible materials;
- The rig substructure, derrick, mast, other equipment, and caravans grounded to prevent accumulation of static charges;
- All equipment or machines (including escape and guy lines) to have minimum clearance of 10ft of power line plus 4 inches for each additional 10 KV over 50 KV or the power lines deenergized and visibly grounded or barriers present to prevent physical contact with the lines;
- Muster area designated and clearly posted with directional signs;
- Access control and visitors tracking system;
- Emergency response alarms available;

- Hazardous locations identified;
- Good housekeeping;
- Electricity generators located a minimum distance of 100 ft (30.5 m) from the well bore.

4.3 Drilling Ahead

Drilling ahead is the common parlance for the actual drilling of the well. This involves a lot of activities like: handling tubulars; preparation of drilling muds; starting the drilling process; breaking out pipe; making up pipe in the 'mousehole'; adding pipe to the string; tripping out/in and coring.

The potential hazards are: being struck by falling or rolling tubulars; hazardous materials (drilling mud); being struck by spinning or swinging tools (like chains, tongs, kelly etc.); loose clothing or body part being caught in rotating equipment; electricity; being thrown off rotary table; shallow gas; slips, trips and falls; noise; falling from heights; high pressure.

To eliminate or minimize the risk posed by these hazards, the safety rules and requirements are typical of those in materials handling, use of forklifts, hazardous materials (all explained in chapter 2), lifting, machine guarding, fall protection and electrical equipment (all explained in chapter 5).In addition, the following should be in place in the following areas:

> ➤ **Mud Pump, Mixing and Mud Tanks/Pits Areas**

- Adequate personal protective equipment (rubber gloves, apron, face shield, goggles, respirators, full and half face mask, safety shoes, hard hats, coveralls) available and used by employees.
- "PPE Required" warning signs erected (specifying the required PPEs).
- Material safety data sheet (MSDS) for the chemicals in use.
- Emergency eye wash and safety shower station available within 10 seconds walking distance and functional, with safety instructions.
- Area with adequate ventilation and lighting.
- Drive belts, chains, gears, shafts and all moving parts adequately guarded.
- End of relief lines (in the mud pump area) located and anchored so as to prevent harm to people due to sudden discharge.

- High pressure rigid lines and tools appropriately secured to prevent movement and harm should they fail.
- Pressures relieve valve installed in the mud pump and has valid testing date.
- Pumps, piping, hoses, valves and other fittings should not be operated at pressures exceeding their rated pressures.
- Guardrails and handrails erected where people could fall from height.
- Shale shaker motor, fixtures, wirings and all equipment within 5 ft (1.5m) of the motor area shall be explosion proof.
- Electrical wiring in good condition.

➤ Hoisting Tools, Hooks, Bails, Elevators and Related Equipment

- Hoisting tools/lines, hooks, bails, elevators and related equipment should be regularly inspected in line with the inspection schedule and defective or missing parts replaced. The schedule should be based on the manufacturer's recommendations, experience, environment, load cycles, regulatory requirements, and operating time.
- Hoisting hooks should have safety latches in order to prevent loads being accidentally released.
- Travelling blocks should be properly guarded and should never be operated without the guards in place.
- Crown block assemblies should be adequately secured in order to prevent the sheaves from jumping out of bearings.
- While being lubricated, travelling blocks should not be moved.

➤ Drawworks

- A visual inspection of the drawworks guard should be made at least once a day (to ensure it is in place and in good condition).
- Drawworks brake systems should be inspected and properly maintained according to the manufacturer's recommendations.
- There should be a safety device designed to prevent the travelling block from striking the crown block. This device should be tested before each trip and after each drill-line slipping/cutting operation and results properly documented.

- The drawworks operator should always be at or near the controls while in operation.

➢ **Drill Floor Area**

- The rotary table power should not be engaged until cleared of personnel and materials.
- The guard on the rotary chain should be inspected daily and confirmed to be in place.
- The weight indicator should have valid calibration.
- Pipe slips and dies in good condition.
- Cathead friction surface and catline divider/grip in good conditions.
- Adequate and explosion proof lighting installed.
- Drill floor maintained clean and free of debris and tripping hazards.
- Means provided to convey any fluids away from the rig floor. Leaks or spills promptly cleaned up to eliminate personnel slipping and fire hazards.
- First aid kit in drill floor doghouse.
- All unused floor holes either covered or guardrails installed.

4.4 Casing Operations

Casing is a larger diameter pipe that is used to line the hole in order to prevent the wall of the hole from caving in, prevent movement of fluids from one formation to another and help in well control. Casing operations involve running and cementing strings of casing in accordance with the design requirements of the well.

The activities involved in casing operations are generally the following: Installing casing tools; running casing into the hole; installing casing accessories; circulation and cementing. The potential hazards and controls are similar to those for Drilling Ahead.

4.5 Well Control

Well control is the management of the unexpected release of formation fluid, such as gas and/or crude oil upon surface equipment of the drilling rig and escaping into the atmosphere. It involves preventing the formation fluid, usually referred to as kick, from entering into the wellbore during drilling. Failure to manage this can cause blowouts, which are uncontrolled and explosive expulsions of formation fluid from the well, potentially resulting in a fire, loss of the rig and other equipment, injury or loss of life.

The primary method of well control uses the mud weight to provide sufficient pressure to prevent an influx of formation fluid into the wellbore. Safety in the operation of the mud system has already dealt with inSection 4.3 (Drilling Ahead).

The secondary method of well control uses the blow-out preventer (BOP). BOP is a large valve at the top of a well that could be closed if control of formation is lost. When this valve is closed (usually remotely via hydraulic actuators), the drilling crew regains control of the reservoir and then some procedures can be initiated to vary the mud density until it is possible to open the BOP and retain control of the formation. The following should be in place to ensure the BOP functions effectively:

- BOP tested and determined to be serviceable before the commencement of drilling operation;
- BOP (while in service) inspected daily and actuation test performed on each round trip (but not more than once in 24 hours) and documented;
- BOP stack and riser connections not short bolted (no less than three threads showing) and the bolts properly torque;
- All hydraulic lines well secured to prevent whipping if pressure surges and all unused lines capped and secured as well;
- The accumulator unit properly located, accumulator bottles correctly labelled, and accumulator operation warning signs erected;
- Safety (stabbing) valve and handle for tubing installed;
- All BOP control lines and valves properly identified.

Where the formation cannot be controlled by primary or secondary well control, the tertiary method is put in place. This involves the drilling of a relief well through which heavy mud is pumped to kill the troublesome well.

4.6 Perforating Operations

In a perforating operation, perforating guns (loaded with explosive charges) are lowered into the well on an electrical wireline to the required depth and electrically activated to fire and create holes in the casing. In addition to following the directions recommended in Use of Explosives (chapter 3), the following should also be in place during perforating operations.

- Non-essential internal combustion engines and equipment that could constitute sources of ignition should be shut down during perforating operations.
- Good communication system between all personnel carrying out the operations should be deployed.
- Electrical grounding between wellhead, service unit and rig structure should be done prior to perforating.
- Strict access control should be enforced during the operations.
- Perforating guns should be assembled in a restricted area designated as such. This area should be free of potential activation sources such as electrical devices, and stray current.
- Radios and mobile phones should be turned off during perforating operations and there should be a warning sign specifying that.
- Perforating operations should not be performed in lightning or stormy weathers and in the night.
- Instruments for testing blasting devices should be specifically designed and labeled as such.
- Conductor wire and armor of perforating gun should be temporarily shorted prior to use.

4.7 Generator Area and Electrical Systems

Generators are used to power equipment and provide lighting on the rig, office and accommodation. The following minimal safety requirements are advised to ensure that they are operated safely.

- On land rigs, electricity generators should be placed at least 100 ft (30.5 m) from the wellhead upwind of the prevailing wind direction.
- Generators should have overload safety device to provide protection from shorting and burnout.
- Electrical extension cords should be well insulated and plugs not damaged.

- Lighting and fixtures should be the appropriate electrical classification for the area it is installed.
- Maintenance work should not be carried out on electrical equipment unless it is properly isolated, locked-out and tagged-out.
- Electrical equipment should be properly grounded.
- Emergency shut-down devices should be installed on all diesel generators (and any other diesel engines).
- Rig power emergency shut-down devices should be actuation-checked at least once a week to determine they are functional.
- All electrical controls should be legibly marked as to their function.
- Electrical wiring should be properly secured and not constitute tripping hazard.
- Moving parts should be guarded.

4.8 Drilling Over Water

When drilling operations is being conducted over water, the following measures should be in place.

- All personnel should be trained in swimming and certified to have capability to swim to personal survival.
- Emergency response procedures (with respect to water operation) should be developed, well resourced and communicated to all personnel on the rig.
- A minimum of two emergency escape means should be available.
- Personal Floatation Devices (PFD) should be provided for all personnel and in serviceable condition.
- Ring buoys with lines should be available and kept in strategic positions.
- There should be a minimum of two approved life boats and each should be capable of accommodating all personnel on board the rig.
- A basket stretcher shall be provided, maintained in an accessible place and inspected at frequent intervals. It should also be used exclusively for transporting injured or sick people and never be used for transferring materials, tools or equipment.
- During helicopter landing and takeoff, crane operations should be suspended.

Chapter 5

CONSTRUCTION, OPERATION
AND MAINTENANCE

5.1 Excavation and Trenching

Excavation and trenching are considered to be some of the most hazardous activities in the petroleum and construction industries. Excavation is any man-made cavity, cut or depression formed by earth removal from the earth's surface. A trench is a narrow underground excavation that is deeper than it is wide and not wider than 15 feet (4.5 meters).

Some of the potential hazards posed by excavation and trenching are as follows: cave-ins (or excavation collapse); fall of adjacent structures; fall of personnel and mobile equipment into excavation; damage to underground facilities like water, gas, and oil pipelines, electricity and telecommunication cables; and hazardous atmospheres.

Excavation and trenching activities should be properly planned and executed under the supervision of a competent person. Prior to the commencement of the activity, the competent person should evaluate the following:

- Size of the excavation and purpose;
- Soil type and stability;
- Proximity and condition of adjacent structures (buildings, scaffolds, roads, railways, equipment etc);
- Proximity of overhead power lines;
- Heavy equipment working nearby;

- Underground facilities like water pipelines, gas/oil pipelines, underground electric/communication cables;
- Nearby hydrocarbon or hazardous materials process facilities;
- Method of excavation, mechanical or manual;
- Method of cave-in protection;
- Location of barricades and warning signs;
- Means of entry and exit from the excavation;
- Means of rescue of personnel from excavation if injured or ill;
- Route of emergency response vehicles to the site or other nearby facilities.

In order to minimize or eliminate the risks of hazards in excavation, the following measures are required to be considered and implemented:

- Excavations 5 feet (1.5 meters) deep or more should be protected from cave-in unless the excavation is made entirely in stable rock. If the depth is up to 20 feet (6.1 meters), the protective system should be designed by a registered professional engineer or be based on tabulated data prepared and/or approved by a registered professional engineer. Protective system could either be shoring or the sides benched or sloped back to a safe angle. Depending on the nature of the soil, these systems could also be combined.

Figure 8: Methods of Excavation Protection

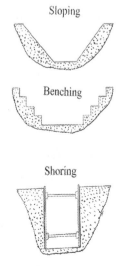

Sloping

Benching

Shoring

- All underground facilities should be identified and appropriate operators notified of the proposed excavation activities before commencement. The locations of the facilities should be reviewed with the operator, appropriate precautions agreed on and implemented to ensure damage or contact does not occur. Mechanical excavators should not be used within 10 feet (3 meters) of any underground facility.
- Personnel should not be inside the excavation when mechanical equipment is being used. In addition, heavy equipment should not be operated within 6 feet (1.8 meters) of any excavation. Cranes should not be operated closer than the depth of the excavation (meaning, if for example the depth of the excavation is 1 meter, cranes should not be operated closer than 1 meter). Barricades, guard rails, warning signs (including blinking lights in the night) should be erected at safe distances to warn people and mobile equipment above the excavation (especially if left unattended).
- Excavated earth or spoils should not be heaped closer than 2 feet (0.6 meters) from the edge of the excavation.
- Support systems should be provided to stabilize adjacent structures, buildings, roadways, sidewalks, etc. The support systems should be installed without exposing employees to cave-ins, collapses or "struck-bys". The base of scaffolds away from the edge of an excavation should be at least 1.5 times the depth of the excavation.
- Precautions should be taken to protect employees from water accumulation (if need be) by continuous dewatering. Surface water or runoff should be diverted or controlled to prevent accumulation in the excavation. The site should be inspected after every rainstorm or other hazard-increasing occurrence.
- Air in the excavation should be tested for oxygen deficiency, combustibles and other hazardous contaminants (like hydrogen sulfide). This test should be conducted prior to entry of personnel and at pre-determined intervals. The testing equipment should have valid calibration, be function-tested on a daily basis and test records properly documented. Mechanical ventilation should be deployed in atmospheres that are oxygen rich/deficient and/or contains hazardous substances.

- Exit ladders should be provided no further than 25 feet from any employee inside the excavation. The ladders should be secured and extend 3 feet above the edge of the excavation.
- Emergency rescue equipment should be available on site in case an employee gets injured or falls ill inside the excavation (especially where hazardous atmospheres could or do exist). Safety harness, lifeline and winch could be used.
- At the start of every shift, a competent person should inspect the excavation with an approved checklist to ensure that all safety measures are in place, adequate and functional. The daily inspection report should be documented.

5.2 Work at Heights

Work at heights remains one of the leading causes of fatalities and serious injury. 'Work at height' means work in any place where, without adequate precautions in place, a person could fall a distance capable of causing personal injury or even death. Work at heights should be properly planned, supervised and carried out by competent people with the skills, knowledge and experience to do the job. The risk should first be assessed and the following factors weighed: the height of the task; the duration and frequency; and the condition of the surface being worked on.

Before working at height it is important to work these simple steps:

- Avoid work at height where it is reasonably practicable to do so;
- Where work at height cannot be easily avoided, prevent falls using either an existing place of work that is already safe or the right type of equipment;
- Minimize the distance and consequences of a fall, by using the right type of equipment where the risk cannot be eliminated.

The following are safe methods of working at heights:

o Personal Fall Arrest Systems

A personal fall arrest system is one option of protecting personnel if the working height is greater than 6 feet (1.8 meters) from grade. It is comprised of three (3) key components – anchorage/anchorage connector; body wear; and connecting device.

Anchorage/Anchorage Connector – anchorage is commonly referred to as a tie-off point (examples: lifeline, I-beam, rebar, scaffolding) and anchorage connector is the connecting device to the anchorage (examples: cross-arm strap, beam anchor, D-bolt, hook anchor). An anchorage should be capable of supporting 5,000 pounds of force per worker. It should be high enough for a worker to avoid contact with a lower level should a fall occur. And the anchorage connector should be positioned to avoid a "swing fall".

Body wear is the personal protective equipment worn by the worker. In the petroleum industry, the only form of body wear acceptable by many companies for fall arrest is the full-body harness.

Connecting Device – this is the critical link which joins the body wear to the anchorage/anchorage connector. Examples are shock-absorbing lanyard, fall limiter, self-retracting lifeline, and rope grab. The potential fall distance should be calculated in order to determine the type of connecting device to be used. For distances under 18.5 feet (5.6 meters), self-retracting lifeline/fall limiter should be used. Shock-absorbing lanyard or self-retracting lifeline/fall limiter should be used when the height is over 18.5 feet (5.6 meters).

When using personal fall arrest systems, the following measures are important:
- Users should inspect the device prior to each use and defective components discarded.
- The components of the device should be protected against cuts or abrasions and should not be used to hoist materials.
- A device should not be used after stopping a fall as the components could have weakened.

Figure 9: Worker Wearing Personal Fall Arrest Equipment

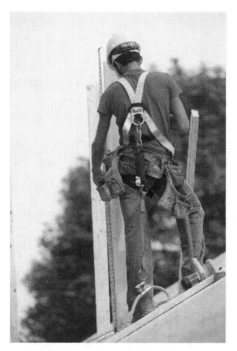

o Scaffolds

Scaffold is a temporary work platform used to support personnel and materials when working at height. Scaffolds should be properly designed, erected and inspected by competent and certified personnel.

There are various types of scaffolds and some of them are: supported, suspended, tower and mobile scaffolds. The most commonly used form is the supported scaffold that is built from the base upwards. The standard components are as follows:

- Sole boards – these support the scaffold post on soft surfaces to ensure it does not sink and loose balance.
- Base plate- these are installed below the posts, sometimes with screw jacks, if there is a need to even out the level.
- Post – these are the vertical standards that support the scaffold structure.
- Bearers- these the horizontal supports that run across the width of the scaffold and on which the working platform rests.

- Runners – these are the horizontal supports of the working platform that run along the length of the scaffold. The bearers rest on top of the runners.
- Planks (boards) – these form the working platform.
- Toe board – these rests on the working platform at all open ends to prevent materials from falling on top of people below.
- Longitudinal bracing & transverse bracings - these keep the scaffold structure stable.
- Top rail – this is the horizontal guard rail installed at the height of between 38 and 45 inches (0.95 – 1.15 meters) above the working platform.
- Mid rail - this is the horizontal guard rail installed midway between the top rail and the working platform.
- Access and egress Ladder – this is installed for safe access and egress from the platform.

Scaffolds should be erected by personnel trained and competent in erecting scaffolds. The erection should be supervised by experienced and competent scaffold supervisors. During and after the erection of a scaffold, it should be appropriately tagged by a certified and authorized scaffold inspector. Before using a scaffold it is important to check the components are complete and that it is tagged. A scaffold tag gives its safety status. Scaffold tags come in three colors: green, yellow and red. A green tag indicates that the scaffold is safe for use within the validity period indicated on it. The tag will also specify the maximum allowable load. A scaffold that is past its validity date should not be used until it has been re-inspected. A yellow scaff-tag indicates it is not safe to use without a personal fall arrest system within the specified validity period. A scaffold without a tag or with a red scaf-tag should not used.

The simple tips for the safe use of a scaffold are as follows:

- It should be inspected each day (using an approved checklist) before use to ensure it has the correct tag and that it has not been tampered with.
- No part of the scaffold should be removed; otherwise it must be re-inspected by a certified person.
- It should not be loaded beyond the capacity specified on the tag.

- It should be re-inspected after every rain or heavy wind.
- Personnel should not climb the braces but use the ladders.
- Unsafe areas underneath the scaffold should be roped-off to prevent passers by being hit by falling objects.
- If it is not practicable to rope off the areas underneath, wire mesh should be provided around the work area.

o Elevating Work Platforms

An elevating work platform (EWP) is a mechanical device that provides a safe platform when working at heights. Scissor lifts, cherry pickers, boom lifts and travel towers are all types of EWPs. They can be battery powered or make use of internal combustion engines.

The safety tips required to work with EWP are as follows:

- Only qualified and authorized personnel should operate EWPs.
- Pre-start up check should be performed on EWP at least once every day and documented.
- EWP should not be operated closer than 10 feet (3 meters) to power lines with voltage up to 50KV; 20 feet (6 meters) for voltages between 50 KV and 250KV; and 25 feet (7.5 meters) for voltages above 250 KV.
- Personal fall arrest devices should be worn at all times while inside EWP.
- Personnel should never enter or leave EWP when it is elevated and should remain within the confines of the work platform at all times.
- Personnel should not stand on the handrails of the platform.
- EWP should not be used as a crane or hoist and materials should not be slung or attached to the side of a EWP, unless the attachment has been specifically designed, rated, tested, marked and approved by the manufacturer of the EWP.
- EWP should not be operated on uncompacted ground.
- Outriggers should always be used in EWP that have them.
- Emergency descent switches should be identified and tested prior to operation.
- Ground controls and descent valves should be known by all personnel.

o Ladder Safety

When the work at height is short time in nature and does not require much physical exertion, it may be advisable to use a ladder, provided the following controls are in place:

- Employees should complete inspection of the ladder and ensure that it is in good condition before each use.
- If it is possible, use only ladders that are Underwriter's Laboratory approved (will have UL seal).
- Ladders should not be painted as paints can hide defects.
- Step ladders should be fully opened and locked before climbing.
- Ladders should be placed on flat, secure, hard and non-movable surfaces.
- It should not be placed in front of a door.
- The base should be positioned one foot away for every four feet of height to where it rests (1:4 ratio) and be properly secured at the top.
- The rails should extend at least three feet above top landing.
- If work is to be done at a height more than 6 feet (1.8 meters) above the ground or working surface, scaffold or EWP should be used instead.
- Before climbing, shoes should be checked to ensure they are free of grease, mud or anything that could cause slippage.
- Users should face the ladder when ascending or descending and ensure at least three points of contact with hands and foot at every moment.
- Tools should be carried in pockets or bags attached to a belt or raised and lowered by rope.
- Do not climb higher than the third rung from the top.
- While working, the user should face the ladder.
- User should not overreach, but always keep his/her torso between the ladder rails.
- It should not be used outdoor on windy days.
- Metallic ladders should not be used around electrical conductors or equipment.
- Only one person is allowed on top of a ladder at a time.

5.3 Work With Cement and Concrete

Cement comprises 7 to 15 percent of total concrete volume. Cement is an alkaline material and caustic when wet. When exposed to skin and eyes cement can cause severe chemical burns. In addition to the caustic nature of cement, 95 percent of cement particles are very tiny and easily inhaled if exposed. Hence working with cement and fresh concrete presents obvious risks and the following safety measures should be followed:

- Always wear rubber hand gloves, long sleeved shirt, full-length trousers and proper eye protection.
- If you have to stand in wet concrete, use rubber boots that are high enough to keep concrete from flowing into them.
- Eye wash and safety shower units should be readily available where concrete work is being done.
- If personnel have skin contact with wet concrete, mortar, cement or cement mixtures it should be washed away immediately.
- Eyes should be flushed with clean water immediately after contact.
- Indirect contact through clothing can be as serious as direct contact so it is important to promptly rinse out wet concrete, mortar, cement or cement mixtures from clothing.
- Always seek immediate medical attention if you have persistent or severe discomfort.
- Workers opening bags or sacks of cement and cement products should always wear a dust mask.

5.4 Lifting and Hoisting

Lifting and hoisting operations are one of the leading causes of fatalities and serious incidents in the petroleum industry. Every type of lift needs to be properly planned and executed subject to the requirements of local legislation in order to minimize or completely eliminate the risk they pose.

Planning the Lifting Operation

Every lift should have a plan, identifying the hazards, analyzing the risks and putting control measures in place. This can be a stand-alone document or part of other documents, the details varying with the risk and complexity of the lift. Simple and routine lifts may only require a generic plan, with an onsite risk assessment and pre-job tool box meeting. Critical lifts may require engineering design input, with drawings and calculations. A lift plan should be approved by a competent person.

A lift should be considered critical if:

- It is within 35 feet (10 meters) of hydrocarbon facility/equipment/ piping, or pressurized equipment/piping or populated/traffic areas or railway line or the fully extended boom of the lifting equipment is within 35 feet (10 meters) of overhead power lines;
- The load is 40 tons or greater;
- The load exceeds 90% of the lifting equipment rated load capacity;
- The load has potential for explosion/fire/high heat hazard;
- It is a tandem lift (i.e. requiring two equipment to lift same load);
- The load is a man-basket;
- The lifting operation is conducted in the night;
- It is a blind lift (i.e. the load is not within sight view of the equipment operator at any point during the operation).

The lift plan should address and specify the following (as a minimum):

- The nature and weight of the load and lifting points;
- Equipment and rigging hardware required and certification checks;
- The type and number of personnel required, their roles and competencies;
- Pick up and set down points and constraints (if any);
- Step-by-step instructions;
- Means of communication;
- Emergency response plans;
- Environmental condition - weather, lighting, sea state(if on water) etc.;
- Access and egress routes for slinging and un-slinging the load;
- Concurrent or nearby operations (and type of work permit, if required);
- Load integrity checks;
- Load charts;
- Assessment of necessity to use tag lines, checking any additional hazards.

Conducting the Lifting Operation

One competent person (a rigger) should be designated as the person in charge of the lifting operation and he should be at the site at all times while the activity is ongoing. The following should be his responsibilities:

- Coordinates, controls and executes the lift;
- Reviews the lift plan and ensures that each of the controls specified is in place;
- Inspects the lifting equipment and rigging hardware to ascertain they are appropriate and safe for use;
- Ensures that the equipment operator and any other person involved are competent, aware of the procedures to be followed and their responsibilities.
- Communicates the lift plan to all the people involved;
- Communicates the activity to nearby work crew and any other people that may be affected;
- Ensures the lift is carried out in line with the approved lift plan and suspends the operation if changes not envisaged in the plan takes place (for example, change in wind speed or direction);

The required competence for equipment operator, rigger and other people involved in lifting operation should be specified by local legislation.

While conducting the lifting, the following critical practices should be followed:

- Before starting lifting operations the rigger in charge of the lift should hold pre-job meeting to communicate the lift plan to all involved.
- When lifting operations is to be controlled by hand signals, a signal man should be designated and possibly wear peculiar reflective jacket.
- The signal man should be trained and competent for the job.
- The hand signal to be used should be the universal signal understood by everybody.
- When radio communication is to be used, continuous verbal instruction shall be used and the operator should stop when there is no clearly understood signal or instruction.
- The lifting equipment operator should obey an emergency stop signal at all times, no matter who gives it;

- The lifting equipment and rigging hardware shall be rated for the load being lifted;
- The safe working load of the lifting equipment and rigging hardware should be clearly marked on them;
- The equipment maintenance records and certification should be readily available and verifiable on site;
- Lifting equipment and rigging hardware should undergo detailed/ thorough examination by a competent person at least once a year (half-yearly if used to lift people);
- The lifting equipment should be inspected and documented on daily basis to ensure the safety devices are in place and functional. Defective components should be repaired before the equipment is put to use.
- Rigging hardware that have been examined and approved to be used within the year should be colored coded. The approved color code for every period should be communicated to all personnel. For example, if in the year 2015, it could be specified that the color code is GREEN. The color code should be displayed on the notice board and communicated to all personnel. For that year 2015, all rigging hardware that have been examined and approved for use will be color-coded GREEN (by application of the color in a conspicuous part of the hardware). However, the user should visually inspect the hardware before each use. Any defective hardware should be discarded immediately
- The equipment operator should not leave the operating controls while the load is suspended;
- Each personnel involved in the lifting operation should not undertake more than one activity at a time;
- Strict access control should be enforced where lifting operations is being undertaken. The work area, including the swing radius should be demarcated with barrier tape and warning signs erected. No one should work or be under a lifted load. Loads should not be moved directly above people.
- Personnel should have escape routes in case of emergency.
- Out riggers should be used (with pads) as per manufacturer's specification.

5.5 Work Permit System

Work permit system is a formal and documented process used to control work that is identified as non-routine or potentially hazardous. It ensures that the activity has been properly planned, consideration given to the risks involved and that all concerned parties have been communicated. When a permit is issued, it authorizes certain people to carry out specific work, at a certain time, at a specific facility or place, using specific equipment and sets out the main precautions required to complete the work safely.

Each organization or company should develop its own work permit procedure but the essential features of the system are:

- Identification of types of work considered as non-routine and potentially hazardous, and facilities applicable;
- Clear roles and responsibilities (identifying who may authorize specific types of jobs, who is responsible for specifying precautions, who is responsible for checking the work site before and after, etc.);
- Training in the issue, use and closure of work permits;
- Monitoring and auditing to ensure that the system is being implemented as required.

Work permits should be considered whenever:

- the proposed job is non-production (for examples, maintenance, repair, inspection, testing, construction, dismantling, assembling, cleaning, modification, adaptation, etc);
- the activities are in a facility specified in the organization's work permit procedure, non-routine and require some kind of job safety analysis;
- two or more different set of crews or different contractors are in a site or facility conducting different jobs and need to co-ordinate their activities to ensure that their work is completed safely.

It should however not be used for activities considered as low risk so as not to trivialize it thereby weakening the overall effectiveness.

Responsibilities – In an organization's work permit system, the following individuals should have specific responsibilities defined in the Work Permit procedure.

Employers or duty holder or installation owner or company chief executive should ensure:

- an appropriate work permit system is developed;
- adequate resources to implement the system is provided;
- training programs and competence standards to implement the work permit system are established and maintained;
- Monitoring, auditing and review of the system are established and maintained.

The facility manager should ensure that:

- All work and facilities requiring work permit are identified and specified;
- Personnel who have roles in the administration of work permit have the competence specified in the procedure;
- The administration of work permit in his area of responsibility is properly coordinated;
- The system is monitored and audited to ensure effective implementation.

Contractor's and sub-contractor's management should ensure that:

- They are aware of and understand the work permit procedure for the locations where their employees are to work;
- Their employees have the competence specified in the procedure, understand the operation of the system and their specified responsibilities within it;
- They have adequate resources to implement the system.

Permit issuer or operations supervisor of the specific unit where the work is to be carried out should have sufficient knowledge about the hazards associated with the plant, and be able to specify control measures correctly. He should ensure that:

- The nature of the work is clearly specified and understood;
- All associated hazards are correctly identified and necessary precautions are in place before commencement of work (including isolation of energy sources and gas testing);
- The permit receiver (or person in charge of the work) has the competence specified in the procedure to fulfill his responsibilities;
- Everybody who may be affected by the activity are informed and kept in the communication loop until the work is completed;
- There is a joint site inspection prior to issuing and close-out of the permit;
- Site is monitored throughout the duration of the work to ensure that the necessary precautions remain in place or otherwise withdraw the permit and stop the job;
- If the work extends beyond his shift, that there is effective handover to the supervisor of the next sheet;
- Keep copies of issued work permits for the period specified by local legislation.

Permit receiver (or person in charge of the work), whether employed by the employer, duty holder or contractor, should ensure that:

- He and his crew have the competence specified in the work permit procedure to fulfill their respective responsibilities;
- The scope of the job is discussed fully with the permit issuer;
- Joint inspection of the site is conducted with the permit issuer to ensure that all necessary precautions are in place (including isolation of energy sources and gas testing);
- His crew is briefed on the details of the permit, potential hazards and necessary precautions;
- All precautions are in place throughout the duration of the work;
- On completion or suspension of the work the facility is made safe, and joint site inspection conducted before closure of the permit and hand back to the issuer.

Work Permit Types and Forms – The center of the work permit system is the paper or electronic form that is used in facilitating communication between all the people involved. Every company or organization that needs to operate the system should design its own forms for the different types of work permits and every effort should be made to keep it simple and user friendly.

The essential contents of the form should be the following:

- Permit type
- Permit number
- Identity of the facility/plant/equipment where the work will be done
- Exact work location
- Description of work to be done
- Details of equipment and tools to be used for the work
- Details of potential hazards
- Precautions necessary and actions in the event of emergency
- Details of protective equipment to be used
- Required gas tests, frequency and records
- Other persons to be notified or countersign
- Date of work and period of validity
- Signature of permit issuer
- Signature of permit receiver
- Signature of gas tester
- Signature of handover of responsibilities between shifts
- Extension of permit after the validity period
- Signature of issuer and receiver to close out permit.

The forms should be colored-coded as to the types of permits so as to be able to differentiate one from the other. The following are the suggested types of work permits and color coding of the forms:

- Hot Work Permit – hot work permit should be used when the type of work to be done can be a source of ignition, the equipment to be used or the work activity itself can generate sparks, flames, and heat that could ignite materials. Examples are welding, flame cutting, use of grinders, abrasive blasting, use of internal combustion engines. Hot work permit forms could be colored red.
- Cold Work Permit – cold work permit should be used when the work will not produce sufficient energy to cause an ignition. Examples could be masonry work, excavation with hand tools. The color could be blue.

- <u>Confined Space Entry Permit</u> – confined space entry permit could be colored green and should be used when the work involves entry into a place that is considered a 'confined space'.
- <u>Breakage of Containment Permit</u> – breakage of containment permit should be used when the work involves breaking open a vessel, equipment or pipeline that has the potential to contain flammable, explosive, hazardous or high pressure fluid. The form could be colored yellow.
- <u>High Voltage Electrical Work Permit</u> – high voltage electrical work permit should be used when the work involves high voltage electrical equipment or conductors. The form could be colored orange.

Whether the forms are in hard copy or electronic based, it is very essential that the use of each type is understood by everyone involved in the activity.

Competence and Training – A work permit system is only as good as the competence of the people who operate it. The employer's chief executive (or duty holder), facility manager, contractors & sub-contractors management, permit issuers and receivers should have sufficient knowledge of the system.

In addition, work permit issuers/receivers should be in supervisory positions and should be competent in their respective professions or trade. The issuer should have sufficient knowledge of the facility in which he is working, viz: plant and equipment layout; the process (production or drilling); potential hazards existing; means to control the hazards in order to make the facility safe for the work to be done; required actions in case of emergency; and company safety rules/procedures.

Both the issuer and receiver should attend training on the requirements of the work permit system, which should include:

- Local legislation and company policy on work permit system
- Industry guidance and case histories of incidents whose root causes are failure of work permit systems
- Gas testing and monitoring
- Basics of hazard recognition and job safety analysis
- Safety requirements for work in confined spaces
- Isolation procedures, lock out and use of hold tag
- Employer's work permit procedure or system

At the end of the training, a written examination should be conducted to assess the level of understanding of the candidates. Those who are successful in the examination should be given certificates and be designated as 'Competent Persons' to issue and receive work permits with respect to their respective areas of trade or profession.

Issuance and Use of Work Permits – When work is to be carried out in facilities where work permit system is applicable:

- the permit receiver (responsible for carrying out the job) and his team should conduct a job safety analysis of the proposed activity;
- the receiver should request a work permit from the issuer, specifying the scope of work and duration (and submitting a copy of the job safety analysis);
- the issuer should go through the scope of work, the job safety analysis and determine the correct type of permit for the proposed work (it is normal for one activity to require two or more types of permits);
- the issuer should verify that the receiver has a valid work permit certification for the type of work to be performed;
- the issuer and receiver should jointly complete the work permit form, specifying precautions as in the job safety analysis (the issuer can put extra precautions with his knowledge of the facility);
- the issuer and receiver should conduct a joint inspection of the site where the work will be done in order to: take note of the state of the facility and possibly any hazards not already identified; conduct gas tests; put isolations in place (if required); and confirm that the facility is safe for the work to start;
- the issuer and receiver should then sign the permits and if a counter-signature is required, obtain such;
- when all relevant signatures have been gotten, the work can start;
- the permit is signed in duplicate (as a minimum), the original being with the issuer and receiver taking the duplicate;
- while work is on-going the receiver's copy should be displayed on site and the issuer's copy displayed on the permit board in the office or control room;

- both the issuer and receiver should be responsible to ensure that the precautions specified in the permit are in place throughout the duration of the work;
- at the end of the validity period, the permit may be extended or closed and a new one issued (depending on the requirements of the company's work permit procedure);
- in a case of shift change, the out-going and in-coming shift permit receivers should conduct joint site inspections, agree that precautions are adequate and sign in designated columns (of both copies of the permit);
- before permit is closed, both the issuer and receiver should conduct joint site inspection and sign-off that the site has been made safe.

Monitoring and Audit of the Work Permit System – work permit system should be monitored continuously to ensure that the permits are correctly issued; precautions specified on them are being complied with and properly closed. Discrepancies should be noted and discussed with all concerned parties.

Implementation of the system should be audited at least annually and findings used to ensure continuous improvement.

5.6 Isolation, Lock-Out and Use of Hold Tags

There are many sources of energy that are potentially hazardous, some of which are electricity, mechanical energy in machines, crude oil and gas under pressure, compressed air, steam, water under pressure and many other fluids. Isolation is a safety procedure which is used in the industry to ensure these sources of hazardous energy are properly shut off to prevent harm to personnel and asset damage when there is need to perform non-routine services (like maintenance or inspection) on a system.

Lock-out is the placement of a lock on the energy-isolating device that physically puts the system in a safe mode. The energy-isolating device can be a switch, circuit breaker, or a valve. Most of devices have loops or tabs that are locked to a stationary item in the de-energized position such that it is safe to carry out maintenance or service without the equipment being re-energized.

Use of hold tags (or tag-out) is a labelling process that should always be used when a lock-out is in place. This involves attaching a label that has information on: plant and equipment numbers; reason for the isolation; time of isolation; name of the authorized person that did the isolation.

In a nutshell, isolation of an equipment or facility for maintenance or servicing cannot be said to be safe unless lock-out and tag-out (LOTO) is also applied.

Lock-out and tag-out (LOTO) steps – the following steps should be used when an equipment or facility needs to be isolated for the purpose of conducting a non-routine maintenance or service:

- Plan for shutdown – the supervisory operations personnel responsible for the equipment should identify which sources of energy are present and should be controlled; and identify the most effective control methods.
- Communicate to operators – the supervisory operations personnel should then communicate the following information to the equipment operators: isolation, lock & tag positions; reasons for the isolation; estimated isolation period; personnel responsible for lock-out/tag-out; personnel to contact for more information.
- Equipment shutdown – if the system is operating, it should be shutdown normally. The controls should be put in the off position and all moving parts verified to have come to a complete stop.
- Isolation from hazardous energy – depending on the type of energy, the following are the methods of isolation:
  o Electrical energy – electrical disconnect switch should be shifted to the off position and locked in that position.
  o Hydraulic or pneumatic energy – either of the four methods should be used depending on the type of work to be carried, viz: close a single block valve, chain and lock the valve in the closed position; for double block and bleed valves, close the double block valves (and chain/lock them in closed positions) and open the bleed valve (and chain/lock it in open position); disconnect the piping; or install blinds.
- Lock-out/tag-out – after the isolation of hazardous energy is complete, the equipment operator should put his own lock/key followed by the crew(s) that are proposed to work on the equipment. To ensure that the

system cannot be inadvertently operated: each lock should have one key; there should be as many locks on the system as there are different crews working on it. For example: one lock for mechanical crew; one lock for electrical crew and one lock for inspection, provided each crew is working under the direction of one person. Locks can only be removed by the authorized persons that installed them.

- Verify Isolation – the system should then be verified to have been properly isolated before starting work. This can be done by either trying to energize the equipment locally or testing the circuitry or checking the pressure/temperature gauges.
- Perform maintenance or service activity for which the isolation is required.
- Remove the lockout and tag-out devices – on completion of the activity, each maintenance or service crew should inspect the site to ensure: all tools, equipment and materials have been removed to safe locations; all personnel are out of the hazardous area and the system is ready to be put back to service. The locks and tags should then be removed in the reverse order they were put (i.e. equipment operator should remove his/her lock after the service teams have removed theirs).

5.7 Entry Into Confined Spaces

A number of people have been killed or seriously injured in confined spaces and these include those doing the actual work and those who try to rescue them in emergencies. A confined space can be defined as any space of an enclosed nature, not normally intended for human occupancy, in which entry, movement within or exit is restricted. Some examples of confined spaces include tanks, vessels, deep excavations, sewers, valve boxes, ductworks, pipes and combustion chambers in boilers. Once any part of the body passes through an opening into a confined space it is considered to be an entry.

Potential Hazards of Confined Space Entry – Some of the potential hazards in confined spaces are: lack of oxygen; presence of hazardous gases, fumes or vapor; presence of liquids and solids which can suddenly fill the space or release gases into it when agitated; fire and explosions from flammable vapors or excess oxygen; residues left in tanks, vessels or pipes that can give off gas, vapor or fume; and high temperature. Some of these hazards may already be present in a confined space prior to personnel entry or may arise from the work activity or lack of proper isolation.

Requirements for Safe Confined Space Entry – Entry and work in confined spaces should be properly planned and executed. Planning involves identifying the hazards present, assessing the risks and determining adequate precautions to take prior to entry. A complete and sufficient assessment will include consideration of the task; the working environment; working materials, tools and equipment; fitness of personnel; and emergency response arrangements.

If an assessment reveals risk of serious injury or fatality, the following should be done: avoid entry to the confined space and rather do the work from outside; where entry cannot be avoided, a safe system of work should be put in place and implemented; and prior to entry, adequate emergency response arrangements should be put in place.

Safe System of Work in Confined Spaces – In a situation where entry into a confined space cannot be avoided, a safe system for working inside the space should be put in place. In order to minimize or eliminate the risks involved, the results of the risk assessment should be a good guide on the required precautions. The following includes some of the features of a safe system of work.

- Dedication of Confined Space Entry (CSE) Supervisor – CSE Supervisor should be dedicated and given the responsibility to ensure that all precautions(from the risk assessment and local requirements) are taken and should be present on site throughout the period that personnel are inside the confined space.
- Personnel Fitness to Work – The personnel should have sufficient experience in the type of work to be carried out and be properly trained on working in confined spaces. Their physical sizes should also be checked putting into consideration the space layout constraints. In addition, they should be medically fit for such jobs, be fit to wear breathing apparatus and should not have claustrophobia.
- Isolation – The equipment to be worked on should be isolated, locked out and tagged out. For hydraulic/pneumatic isolation, the only

method of isolation suitable for personnel entry into a confined space is blinding.

- Cleaning – the enclosure should be properly cleaned to ensure that fumes do not develop from residues while work is being carried out.
- Gas testing – gas testing should be conducted prior to entry to ensure the atmosphere inside the space has sufficient oxygen and free from toxic and flammable vapors. The testing should be carried by a competent gas tester and the gas detector used should have valid calibration. Depending on the result of the risk assessment, it might be necessary to continuously monitor the atmosphere inside the space. Oxygen concentration should be at least 20%; flammable mixtures should be less than 5% of the lower explosive limit (0%, if hot work will be carried out); and hydrogen sulfide should not exceed 10 parts per million.
- Mechanical ventilation – mechanical ventilation may be required to ensure there is adequate supply of fresh air at the right temperature. This is essential where the type of work being done or the equipment used has the potential to generate gases that are hazardous or can displace oxygen.
- Size of manhole – the size of the manhole for the entry and exit of personnel should be checked to ensure it is big enough to allow workers wearing all necessary PPEs to climb in and out with ease and for emergency rescue.
- Provision of special tools and lighting – Where flammable or potentially explosive atmosphere is present, non-sparking tools and explosion-proof lighting should be used. In confined spaces with metallic parts, suitable precautions to prevent electric shock (like use of extra low-voltage equipment and residual current devices and adequate grounding) should be adopted.
- Use of breathing apparatus –breathing apparatus should be provided and used if the air inside the space does have insufficient oxygen (less than 20%), hazardous fumes, gases or vapors.
- Means of communication – there should be an adequate means of communication between the people inside and outside the confined space and to call for help in case of emergency.

- Standby man – a trained standby man should be positioned outside the space to keep watch and communicate with people inside. The standby man should keep a log of all personnel inside. He should call for emergency, when required. The standby man should never go into the space to carry out rescue unless he has the right equipment and has a replacement (as a standby man).
- Means of access and egress – there should be a safe means of access into and egress out of the confined space.
- Emergency response – rescue equipment including lifelines, harnesses, and hoists should be used if the confined spaces are deeper than 6 feet (1.8 meters). Emergency response procedures should be developed, properly resourced and all personnel trained in them.

5.8 Electrical Safety

The incidents that could result from work on or in close proximity to electrical equipment are: electric shock; electrocution (fatal); burns (from heat generated by an electric arc and flame burns from materials that catch fire); and falls (muscle spasm, or startle reaction or force of explosion from an arc flash can cause a person to fall from height); and hearing loss (from the sound of an arc flash). To minimize or eliminate the risk of these incidents, the following measures should be adopted when working on or in close proximity to electrical conductors and equipment:

- Portable cord-and-plug connected equipment, extension cords, power bars and electrical fittings should be inspected for damage or wear before each use. Damaged equipment should be repaired or replaced immediately.
- Extension cords or equipment to be used should be checked to ensure that they are rated for the level of amperage or wattage that they are being used for. Extension cords should not be used in place of permanent installation.
- The correct size of fuse should always be used. Replacement of a fuse with one larger in size has the potential to cause excessive currents in the wiring with consequences of fire.
- Metal ladders should not be used when working on or in the vicinity of live electrical equipment.

- Ground fault circuit interrupters (GFCIs) should be used for all portable electrical tools, temporary wiring and when working in areas that are wet or damp.
- Exposed receptacle boxes should be made of non-conductive materials.
- Circuit breakers and fuse boxes should be clearly labeled (and always updated) as to which equipment they are for, so that quick isolation can be done in case of emergency.
- Personnel should never open or close a disconnect switch while facing it. They should stand to the side, faces turned away from the switch, and operate it with a quick, single motion.
- Use of jewelry or articles of clothing that have exposed metallic components should be avoided while working on or in close proximity to energized electrical equipment.
- Access to panels and circuits breakers or fuse boxes should always be kept clear.
- Arc flash warning signs should be affixed on high voltage equipment designating approach boundaries and the required PPEs.
- When work is to be done on an electrical conductor or equipment, it should be considered energized unless it has been isolated, locked, tagged and verified (for effective isolation).
- Only qualified personnel should be allowed to repair or install electrical equipment.
- If high voltage equipment cannot be effectively isolated before maintenance or service is carried out on it, only personnel that have received adequate training and have the required competence should be allowed to work on them.
- Personnel who work on live high voltage equipment should follow the requirements of the arc-flash hazard warning signs placed on it by wearing the required PPEs, use insulated tools and other safety related precautions.
- When heavy equipment are to work close to overhead power lines, the minimum safe distances should be as follows: up to 33,000 volts, 3 meters (10 feet); 33,000 volts to 275,000 volts, 6 meters (20 feet); above 275,000 volts, 8 meters (27 feet).
- In locations where hazardous gases, vapors or dust are likely or do exist, electrical equipment (including junction boxes) should be explosion proof type.

5.9 Machine Guarding

Moving parts of machines create workplace hazards and have the potential for very serious injuries. The moving parts could be rotating, reciprocating or transversing. Machine guarding helps to protect workers from such preventable injuries. They are required to be provided wherever moving parts of a machine are less than seven (7) feet above the floor or working level and should meet the following minimum general requirements:

- Should prevent hands, arms or any other part of a worker's body from making contact with moving parts.
- Personnel should not be able to easily tamper with or remove the safe guard.
- The safe guards should ensure that objects do not fall into the moving parts.
- They should not create a new hazard such as an unfinished surface, a shear point, or jagged edge.
- The safe guards should not impede workers from getting their jobs done quickly and comfortably so that they do not get tempted into defeating them.
- The machines should be lubricated safely without removing the safe guards.
- Machine guarding materials should be durable and not flammable.
- Guards should be affixed to the machine where possible and secured elsewhere if attachment to the machine is not possible.
- Where a moving part is over seven (7) feet above working level but a failure of such part is assessed to have the potential for harm (like whip lash of a failed belt drive), adequate safe guards should be provided.

5.10 Pressure Testing

Pressure testing is a process of applying stored energy to a facility or equipment (such as pipelines, pressure vessels, boilers, gas cylinders) in order to test its strength, integrity and leaks. It involves filling the equipment with a fluid and pressurizing it to a specified test pressure and checking whether or not the pressure is maintained within a specified period.

Pressure testing is a high risk activity. The high pressure can explode either the equipment under test or the test assembly, creating flying fragments and the test fluid projected under immense force with potential for serious injuries to exposed workers and assets damage.

In order to minimize or eliminate the risks associated with pressure testing, a written safe system of work should be in place, summarizing the hazards and the controls that must be in place before, during and after the test. This safe system of work should provide written instructions to personnel conducting the test to ensure:

- The equipment is safely energized, monitored and the test medium safely evacuated;
- Correct selection of fittings (verifying that hoses, connectors, and other fittings are rated for the test pressure and medium);
- Correct positioning of pressure relieve devices;
- Safe segregation of all components under pressure and access control to the pressure test site (including positioning of warning signs).

In general, the following safety practices should be in place:

- Job safety analysis should be conducted for every pressure testing operation;
- Pressure testing should be supervised by competent personnel;
- All personnel involved in the testing activity should undergo training, highlighting the hazards and control measures;
- The material safety data sheet (MSDS) of the test fluid and all chemicals to be used should be on site and the specified precautions followed;
- Correct PPEs should be worn by all exposed personnel;
- Appropriately rated relieve valve should be installed to ensure that the equipment being tested is not over pressured;
- Components of the equipment not being tested should either be disconnected or positively isolated;
- Only workers involved in the activity should be allowed access to the test site;
- Pressure gauges should be located at a safe distance (at least 100 feet from the facility being tested);
- The test site should be marked, barricaded and warning signs posted at suitable locations;

- Safe distances should be demarcated for workers performing the test;
- The test equipment should be verified to be rated to withstand the test pressure;
- The system under pressure should be depressurized prior to any adjustment or repair works;
- Adequate lighting should be available throughout the testing activity;
- Safety equipment and supplies should be readily available. Examples are emergency spill kit, fire extinguisher, whip checks and first aid kits.

5.11 Painting and Coating

Paints and coatings can be applied either as solids, liquids or aerosols. They are chemicals products and whichever ways they are applied have health, fire and explosion hazards. Workers can be exposed to health hazards by inhalation, ingestion or absorption of the paint and coating materials. The hazards stem from the chemicals used in making the solvents, pigments and primers, the common ones being toluene, xylene, ketones, esters, alcohols, lead, chromium, nickel, cadmium, zinc, epoxy resins and isocyanates. The main health effects from exposure to these chemicals include: eye and skin irritation; respiratory tract irritation; dermatitis; dizziness; nausea/vomiting; heavy metal poisoning. Chronic exposure can cause long term health effects such as nerve, kidney or liver damage.

The major safety concern associated with painting and coating is the combustible and flammable vapors, mist and residues that are created. Potential sources of ignition of these include: open flames; cutting and welding activities; heating units; electrical sparks; static electricity; smoking.

The following safety measures should be in place in order to minimize the risks associated with painting and coating operations:

- If possible, the paint type should be substituted with non-flammable and less toxic types.
- When painting or coating activity is being conducted in spray booths or rooms, adequate ventilation should be in place.
- Mechanical ventilation equipment should be inspected regularly to ensure they function properly.
- When spray painting is being carried out in a place other than in a spray booth, it should be conducted at least 6 meters from anything

that may block ventilation. Otherwise, the site should be adequately ventilated and all sources of ignition should be removed or isolated.

- Adequate measures should be taken to ensure other workers not involved in the painting activity are informed and that they are not exposed to the paint and coating materials.
- Prior to painting and coating activities, the material safety data sheets should be used to train workers on the associated hazards, and recommended control/recovery measures.
- Correct storage, transportation, use and disposal requirements (as specified in the material safety data sheet) should be followed.
- Appropriate personal protective equipment (including respiratory protective equipment) should be worn by all personnel carrying out painting and coating or who are exposed to the materials (as specified in the materials safety data sheet).
- Functional eye wash and safety shower facilities should be available within the vicinity of painting and coating sites and materials storage areas.
- The painting and coating equipment should be effectively grounded.
- There should be adequate safety signs (especially, restricting ignition sources within the painting zone).
- Flammable paint and coating materials should not be applied on hot surfaces.
- Painting and coating jobs should not be carried out up wind of an ignition source; unless there are adequate measures to ensure that flammable vapors do not drift to the ignition source.
- Spray painting booths should be regularly cleaned of residues with non-sparking tools.

5.12 Abrasive Blasting

Abrasive blasting is a process of using compressed air or water to direct a stream of an abrasive material at high velocity to clean an object or surface, to smoothen, roughen, shape the surface, or remove the surface coatings or contaminants. The abrasive materials used can be any of the following: silica sand, garnet sand, nickel slag, coal slag, glass, steel shot, steel grit, dry ice, plastic bead media, sponge and sodium bicarbonate.

The hazards associated with abrasive blasting operation are as follows:

- *Hazardous Dusts:* Inhalation of the hazardous dust particles produced during abrasive blasting can result into respiratory problem, lungs damage and sometimes, heavy metals poisoning.
- *High Pressure:*People around the work area can be exposed to high pressure arising from the compressed air or water being used. Loss of containment has potential for serious injuries that include particles becoming embedded in the skin, eye damage, severe cuts and burns.
- *High noise level:* High noise levels can cause hearing loss if workers and others in the vicinity are unprotected.
- *Improper manual handling:* Manual handling tasks are also involved. If done improperly it can result in strains, sprains, fractures, dislocations, bruises and overuse injuries.
- *Confined Spaces:* If the activity is carried out in a confined space there could be asphyxiation and death.
- *Carbon monoxide:* Carbon monoxide could be inhaled from oil lubricated air compressors used to supply breathing air resulting to death.
- *Hand-arm vibration:* Prolonged exposure to abrasive blasting vibration can damage the nervous system and result in a condition known as vibration syndrome.
- *Heat over exposure*: Use of the required PPE for long periods without adequate rest can result to heat over exposure.
- *Explosive atmosphere:* If explosive atmosphere exist at the work site the friction of the abrasive material and the surface being worked on can become ignition source.
- *Static Electricity:* There could be accumulation of static charges that can shock employees and cause fires and explosions.

In order to minimize the risks posed by these hazards, the following control measures should be in place:

- Use of less toxic abrasive material should always be explored. For example, in some places, the use of silica sand is prohibited.
- Blast operators should be trained in the correct use and hazards associated with the equipment and materials they use.

- Barriers and curtain walls should be used to isolate the blasting operation from other workers. If possible, exhaust ventilation system should be used to capture the produced dust.
- As much as possible, abrasive blasting jobs should be scheduled when the least number of workers are on site and on less windy days in order to prevent the spread of hazardous dust.
- Operators should wear air-supplied hood, type "CE" (NIOSH-approved) while blasting and other workers in the vicinity must wear air-purifying respirators with dust filters.
- Other required PPEs are hearing protection, eye and face protection, hard hat, leather gloves covering forearm, coveralls, apron, and safety shoes.
- High pressure lines should have safety wire installed in every coupling points to prevent separation. The hoses and couplings should be inspected before use for cuts, abrasion and damage. The abrasive blasting nozzle should have a dead man switch that automatically shuts-off the flow of abrasive material if the operator releases control of the switch or nozzle
- Operators should be trained on proper manual handling techniques.
- If the activity is taking place in a confined space, all confined space entry procedures should be in place.
- Breathing air equipment in use should have high efficiency air filters, oil/water traps and in-line carbon monoxide monitoring with an audible alarm (if oil lubricated breathing air compressors are in use).
- Job rotations or more frequent breaks should be practiced in order to reduce the extent and duration of continuous exposure to vibration and heat.
- Gas test should be performed to ensure that flammable gases are not present.
- The blasting equipment and the structure being cleaned should be connected and effectively grounded in order to prevent static charges from accumulating.
- Warning signs and notices should be placed at strategic locations to inform other workers of the activity.
- Eye wash and safety shower stations should be provided in case of accidental exposure.

- Internal combustion engines to be positioned downwind of the breathing air supply compressor to avoid intake of smoke.

5.13 Hand and Power tools

There are five basic safety rules that can help to control hazards associated with the different types of hand and power tools:

- All tools should be kept in good condition with regular maintenance.
- The right tool and the right size should be used for every job.
- Each tool should be inspected for damage before and after use and damaged ones should be removed from service.
- Tools should be operated according to manufacturers' instructions.
- The correct type of personal protective equipment should be used while using tools.

Hand Tools – Hand tools are tools powered manually and they include screw drivers, pliers, hammers, chisels, saws, spanners, wrenches etc. These are so commonly used that people do not think that they pose hazards. However, serious incidents can occur if tool-related hazards are not effectively controlled. The additional safety precautions necessary for the use of hand tools are as follows:

- Workers should be trained in the safe use, maintenance and storage of hand tools.
- Cutting tools must be sharp; dull tools can cause more hazards than sharp ones.
- When using tools like saw blades and knives, they should be directed away from aisle areas and other employees working in close proximity.
- When used for electrical work, handles of tools should be insulated.
- When working in locations where flammable gases exist or are likely to exist, non-sparking tools made of non-ferrous materials should be used.
- The use of 'cheater bar' extensions in spanners, and wrenches should be discouraged.
- Handles of screw drivers should not be subjected to hammer blows.
- The head of hammers should be properly secured by wedges.

- Appropriate personal protective equipment such as safety goggles and hand gloves should be worn while using hand tools.
- Proper housekeeping should be maintained in the workplace to prevent accidental slips with or around dangerous hand tools.

Power Tools – There are five basic types of power tools, differentiated by their power source and they are: electric, pneumatic, liquid fuel, hydraulic and powder-actuated. All power tools should be fitted with guards and safety switches.

To control hazards associated with the use of power tools, workers should follow the following general precautions:

- Tools should never be carried by the cord or hose. Cords or hoses should never be yanked in order to disconnect the tool from the energy source.
- Cords and hoses should be kept away from heat, oil and sharp edges.
- All tools should be switched OFF before connecting them to a power source.
- Isolation and effective lockout from energy source should be done before carrying out any maintenance work tasks or making adjustments on a power tool.
- Power tools should be properly grounded or double-insulated. They should be tested for effective grounding with a continuity tester or a Ground Fault Circuit Interrupter (GCFI) before use.
- The on/off switches should not be bypassed to operate the tools by connecting and disconnecting the power cords.
- Electrical equipment should not be used in wet conditions or damp locations unless it is connected to a GCFI.
- Works should be secured with clamps or vise, freeing both hands to operate a tool.
- Tools should be maintained with care, keeping them sharp and clean for best performance.
- When lubricating and changing accessories, the manufacturers' manual should be followed.
- When operating power tools, good footing and balance should be maintained.

- Loose clothing, ties, jewelry and long hair can become caught in moving parts and hence should be prohibited while working with or in close proximity to power tools.
- All damaged power tools should be removed from service and tagged: 'Do Not Use.'
- The exposed moving parts of power tools (such as belts, gears, shafts, pulleys, sprockets, spindles, drums, flywheels, chains, or other reciprocating, rotating, or moving parts) should be safe guarded. Safety guards should never be removed when a tool is being used.
- Hand-held power tools should be equipped with a constant-pressure switch or control that shuts off the power when the pressure is released.

Electric Tools–the most serious risks associated with the use of electric tools are burns and shocks. The following additional general practices should be followed when using electric tools:

- To protect users from shock and burns, electric tools should have three-wire cord with a ground and be plugged into a ground receptacle, be double insulated or be powered by a low-voltage isolation transformer. Otherwise, double-insulated tools are available that provide protection against electrical shock.
- Electric tools should be operated within their design limitations.
- Hand gloves and appropriate safety shoes should be worn when operating electric tools.
- Electric tools should be stored in a dry place when not in use.
- Work areas should be kept well lit when operating electric tools.
- Cords from electric tools should be kept such that they do not present a tripping hazard.

Pneumatic Tools– the following additional safety precautions should be followed when using pneumatic tools:

- They should be inspected to see that the tools are fastened securely to the air hose to prevent them from disconnecting. A positive locking device or short wire attaching the air hose to the tool should be used and serve as an added safe guard.

- For a hose that is more than half inch in diameter, a safety excess flow valve should be installed at the source of the air supply in order to reduce pressure in case of hose failure.
- Hoses of pneumatic tools should be kept such that they do not present a tripping hazard.
- When using pneumatic tools, a safety clip should be installed to prevent attachments (such as chisels on a chipping hammer) from being ejected during tool operation.
- Pneumatic tools that shoot fasteners and are operated at pressures more than 100 pounds per square inch (6,890 kPa) should be equipped with a special device to keep fasteners from being ejected, unless the muzzle is pressed against the work surface.
- Eye, ear, face, head, hand and foot protections should be worn by personnel working with pneumatic tools.
- Compressed air guns should never be pointed at people.
- Screens should be set up to protect nearby workers from being struck by flying fragments around chippers, riveting guns, staplers or air drills.
- To reduce the extent and duration of continuous exposure to vibration, job rotations or more frequent breaks should be practiced by workers operating jack hammers.

Liquid Fuel Tools – the most serious hazards associated with the use of fuel-powered tools are from the flammable fuel vapors (with the attendant risk of fire/explosion or asphyxiation by exhaust fumes). Hence, adequate care should be taken in the handling, transportation and storage of the fuel. In addition:

- The engine powering the tool should be shut down and allowed to cool before refueling.
- There should be adequate ventilation if liquid fuel tool is being used in a closed area to avoid carbon monoxide inhalation. In the same vein, it should not be positioned upwind of work location in an open area.
- Adequate fire extinguishers should be available at the work location.

Hydraulic Power Tools– The following safety requirements should be in place:

- The fluid used in hydraulic power tools should be fire resistant.
- The specified safe operating pressure for hoses, valves, pipes, filters and other fittings should not be exceeded.
- Hydraulic jacks should have stop indicators and the stop limit should not be exceeded.
- The load limit for jacks should be written on it and should never be exceeded.
- Jacks should never be used to support a lifted load.
- Jacks should be lubricated and maintained regularly. They should be inspected at least once every six months and when subjected to abnormal loads or sent out of the shop for special use, should be inspected before and after.

Powder-Actuated Tools– The safety precautions that should be in place when using powder-actuated tools are as follows:

- Only trained employees should operate powder-actuated tools.
- Users of powder-actuated tools should wear ear, eye and face protection.
- The tool should not be used in an explosive or flammable atmosphere.
- Users should inspect the tool before using it to determine that it is clean, that all moving parts operate freely and that the barrel is free from obstructions and has the proper shield, guard and attachments as specified by the manufacturer.
- The tool should not be loaded unless it is to be used immediately.
- Loaded tool should not be left unattended.
- The tool should never be pointed at people.
- Fasteners should neither be fired at materials that are so soft that the fasteners could pass through to the other side nor at materials that are so hard or brittle that the fasteners might ricochet or the material splatter.
- Alignment guide should always be used when shooting fasteners into existing holes.
- When using a high velocity tool, the fasteners should not be driven more than 3 inches (7.62 centimeters) from an unsupported edge or

corner of material such as brick or concrete. And fasteners should not be placed in steel any closer than half an inch (1.27 centimeters) from an unsupported corner edge unless a special guard, fixture or jig is used.

5.14 Work with Heavy Mobile Equipment

Unsafe use of heavy mobile equipment can result in serious injury, loss of life, or property damage. To eliminate or minimize the risk associated with the heavy mobile equipment:

- Operators should be trained and be licensed by the government on the specific equipment.
- Heavy mobile equipment should be inspected and undergo preventive maintenance on a regular basis in line with the manufacturer's specification by a competent heavy equipment mechanic.
- Prior to the use of all heavy equipment, they should be inspected by the operator. The items to check in the inspection should include: lights, horn, back-up alarm working properly; electrical wirings in good order; hose and pipe connections not worn or cracked; fuel, oil, hydraulic and water not leaking; seat belt in place; functional brakes; fire extinguishers available.
- When undergoing maintenance, equipment operators should not be allowed to be on the equipment, unless there is a need to. Repairs cannot be carried out while the equipment is running.
- Repairs on heavy equipment tires should not be conducted while they are inflated. And they should be inflated inside a tire cage by experienced personnel.
- While operating heavy equipment, the operator should have 360-degree visibility.
- There should be strict access control to sites where heavy equipment is in operation.
- When there are other workers in a site, trained flagmen should be used to help the operator in cases of blind spots. The flagmen should wear reflective vests.

- Diesel- or gasoline-powered heavy equipment should not be used inside buildings or confined spaces to prevent asphyxiation by carbon monoxide from the exhaust.
- When heavy equipment is unattended, the engine should be stopped, parking brake applied and wheels choked. The blades, buckets, scraper bowls and other hydraulic components should be lowered to the ground. In addition, the ignition keys should be removed to prevent unauthorized persons from starting the equipment. If it is to be left unattended overnight, there should be appropriate lights/reflectors, barricades and warning lights, if the area is in a busy construction site or close to a highway.
- While heavy equipment is in operation, personnel should not be allowed to ride on it unless it is so designed.
- Workers should not be allowed to rest or sleep under or around heavy equipment at any time.
- Equipment should not be refueled whilst the engine is running.
- When heavy equipment are to work close to overhead power lines, the minimum safe distances should be as follows: up to 33,000 volts, 3 meters (10 feet); 33,000 volts to 275,000 volts, 6 meters (20 feet); above 275,000 volts, 8 meters (27 feet). Goal posts (corresponding to these heights) should be installed at about 30 meters horizontal distance from the power line to act as guide.

Excavators and backhoes- Additional safety requirements for excavators and backhoes are as follows:

- Workers should not be allowed within the boom radius while an excavator or backhoe is in operation.
- The clearance from the boom radius to any fixed object should be 1 meter (3.3 feet) while performing swinging motion.
- The clearance from the boom radius to any live hydrocarbon facility should be at least 3 meters (10 feet).
- For equipment that is designed with outriggers, these should be fully extended when in operation.
- Excavators should not be used for lifting purposes unless they are so designed.

Graders, Dozers, and Loaders – Additional safety requirements for graders, dozers and loaders are as follows:

- Rollover protection should be provided on graders, dozers and loaders.

Concrete Mixers and Pumping Equipment – Additional safety requirements for concrete mixers and concrete pumping equipment are as follows:

- Respirators, goggles and hearing protection should be worn while working with concrete mixers.
- Moving parts of machines (such as chains, gears, shafts and belts) should be properly guarded.
- Only authorized personnel shall be allowed close to the equipment while in operation.
- There should good housekeeping in the work area.
- A concrete pumping equipment operator should respond to the signal from a designated signal man and to any stop signal from any person.
- A concrete pumping machine should not be used for lifting purposes other than as specified by the manufacturer.
- While a concrete pumping machine is in operation, the outriggers should be fully extended. And when moving, the outriggers should be properly stowed as required by the manufacturer.
- Concrete pumping equipment should not be operated in lightning or when the wind speed exceeds 32 km/hr (20 mph).

Dumpers and Dump Trucks - Additional safety requirements for dumpers and dump trucks are as follows:

- Dumpers and dump trucks should undergo regular preventive maintenance checks and particular attention to be on the brakes, steering and skip release systems.
- Workers should not be allowed to ride in the skip or engine covers of dumpers and dump trucks.
- Dump bodies should be fully lowered before leaving the dump area. They should also be fully lowered when repair or maintenance are being performed. If, however, they are to be in the raised position

for maintenance or any extended period, the dump bodies should be blocked.

- Dumper skip latches and the release mechanism should be in good working order.

5.15 Cutting, Welding and Brazing

The main hazards associated with cutting, welding and brazing are:

- Electric shock
- Overexposure to fumes and gases
- Arc radiation
- Fire, explosion and burns

The following are the safety requirements to ensure that these hazards are controlled:

- Welding equipment should be undergoing regular preventive maintenance checks as recommended by the manufacturers.
- Equipment should be inspected before use on a daily basis and defective ones should be put out of service until the defect is rectified. The following components should be checked: all connections tight; output terminals insulated; electrode holder and welding cables well insulated; and settings correct for the job to begin. For engine-driven machines, is it running ok; are all hoses tight; fuel cap tight; and no fuel or oil leaks.
- Welders should wear proper PPEs that should include flame-resistant clothing, aprons, leggings, leather sleeves/shoulder capes, leather gloves, safety shoes, hard hats and welder's face shield.
- Electric welding machines should be properly bonded and grounded.
- Welding activities should be properly ventilated. When carried out in workshops, mechanical ventilation should be used.
- Welding, cutting and brazing should not be carried out in oxygen enriched atmospheres (concentration greater than 23.5 %).
- There should be good housekeeping around areas where welding, cutting and brazing are being conducted. Combustible materials should be removed and those that cannot be removed should be

covered with fire blankets. Sewers within 25 meters of the welding location should also be covered.

- Portable fire extinguisher should always be available where welding, cutting and brazing operation is being conducted. A trained fire watch should man the extinguisher, watch out to extinguish any incipient fire while the operation is ongoing and at least 30 minutes after. The fire watch should also know how to report fire incidents.
- When flame-cutting or brazing, lighted torches should not be left unattended.
- Oxygen/acetylene cutting sets should be checked before use for leaks (for example, with soap solution).Gauges, regulators, hose, cylinders should be checked for damage and the cylinder should have valid hydro-test date.
- Flashback arrestors should be installed at oxygen and acetylene cylinder regulators. Check valves should be installed at the torch end of the hoses.
- Pressure regulators should have functional gauges.
- Oxygen and acetylene gas regulators should be turned off when not in use.
- Gas hoses should be protected from damage during operations.
- Oxy/acetylene torches should be lit with strikers only.
- Acetylene cylinders should have a handle or valve wrench at all times.
- When attempting to stop gas leaks, the cylinder valve should be closed first.
- Oil or grease should never be used as lubricant on cylinder valves or attachments.
- Gas cylinders should be protected from direct sunlight, flame or any sources of heat.
- Cylinder protective caps should be in place when the cylinders are not in use.
- Cylinders should be transported in upright position, in trolleys or material baskets or cylinder racks or other proper cages. They should never be moved with slings or ropes. While moving cylinders, they should never be knocked on each other.
- In storage, cylinders should be in upright position in cylinder racks.

- Oxygen and acetylene cylinders should not be stored together. There should be at least 20 feet (6.1 meters) separation distance between them. Where such separation distance is not possible, there should be 5 feet (1.5 meter) non-combustible wall between oxygen and acetylene cylinders.
- Stored cylinders should be clearly labeled (empty and full cylinders properly identified).
- Gas cylinders should never be stored at temperatures above 54 degree Celsius (130 degree Fahrenheit).

5.16 Ionizing Radiation

Ionizing radiation is used to investigate the integrity of structures or components through radiographic images, generally referred to as non-destructive radiography or industrial radiography.

Overexposure to ionizing radiation has serious consequences like damage of body cells, leukemia or solid tumor (cancer). In pregnant women, the exposure of the embryo or fetus to ionizing radiation could increase the risk of leukemia in infants, mental retardation, and congenital malformations. The following safety precautions (as a minimum) should be in place to ensure that radiation risk is managed to as low as reasonably achievable (ALARA):

- Procurement, handling, use, storage and disposal of ionizing radiation equipment and consumables is a legal issue and should be conducted in line with local regulation.
- Every ionizing radiation activity should be conducted under the supervision a radiation safety officer (RSO), who should be a certified industrial radiographer (the level of which should be in accordance with the local regulation).
- All industrial ionizing radiation equipment should be registered with the local regulatory authority and the evidence of such registrations should always be available on site.
- No personnel should be allowed to operate ionizing radiation equipment without proper training, licensing and authorization (in line with local regulation).
- Industrial radiographers should be assigned with and wear photon-sensitive passive dosimeters as well as instantaneous reading electronic

alarm dosimeters. Each passive personal dosimeter should be worn by only the individual to whom it has been assigned in order to keep the personnel monitoring data. The data should be retained as a permanent record and be made readily available for review regularly to ensure they do not exceed allowable threshold value.

- As much as possible, radiography should be performed at periods when human traffic is least at the site (most likely in the night).
- Prior to the commencement of radiography, a controlled area should be established. Access into such area should be controlled with barriers, warning signs (visual and audio) and safety instructions strategically posted external to the area. The controlled area should also be monitored by designated individuals to enforce the access restriction.
- Calibrated and functional survey meters should be used to ensure that radiation dose rate at the boundary of the controlled area is within safe limits.
- Temporary radiation control station should be positioned outside the controlled area for the initiation, generation or termination of ionizing radiation and for image acquisition and assessment.
- Personnel who are working in close proximity to the controlled area should be told about the activity, the associated hazards and controlled measures in place.
- Transportation and storage of radioactive sources should be conducted as approved by local regulations in order to prevent undue exposure to the public, theft or loss. Accurate inventory should be kept at all times.
- Conspicuous warning signs should be displayed on vehicles transporting radioactive sources, and at the storage locations.
- Disposal of radioactive waste should also be done in accordance with local regulations.
- Accidents involving radioactive sources or equipment (including theft) should be reported immediately to regulatory authorities and steps taken to give medical attention to any exposed people. Adequate investigation should be conducted to prevent reoccurrence.
- Repair and maintenance of radiation equipment should be carried out only by competent and licensed personnel who should ensure effective isolation is in place before carrying out the job.

5.17 Pile Driving

The potential hazards associated with pile driving are as follows:

- Falling of lifted objects;
- Noise
- Vibration
- Buried or overhead services
- Collapse of nearby structures
- Contact with plant or other equipment during lifting
- Falling from height
- Exposure to high pressure

The safety requirements to have control over these hazards are:

- A method statement should be prepared by a competent supervisor, taking into account the hazards and risks associated with the particular job and all workers on the operation trained in the particular method statement.
- Pile drivers should be properly supported on heavy timber sills, concrete or other firm foundation.
- Pile drivers should be adequately guyed.
- When overhead power lines are in the vicinity of the work location, precautions as prescribed in section 5.8 should be followed.
- All underground facilities should be noted, marked and made safe.
- When two pile drivers are to work on the same location the separation distance should be at least twice the height of the higher pile driver.
- Access to work platforms should be via well secured ladder.
- Couplings of high pressure steam or air hose should be secured by ropes or chains to prevent whiplash if the connection breaks.
- Sheaves on pile drivers should be adequately guarded so that personnel or body parts do not get drawn into them.
- Pile-driving equipment should be inspected before being taken into service and re-inspected at intervals as specified by the manufacturers.
- Before the beginning of each shift the equipment should be inspected, especially the piles and pulley blocks.

- Every repair or maintenance to be done on pile-driving equipment and accessories should be carried out by competent persons. Effective isolation should be in place before the commencement of any maintenance activity.
- Only competent and authorized personnel should be allowed to operate pile drivers.
- Personnel working with or in the vicinity of pile driving equipment should wear hard hats, safety shoes, hand gloves, safety glasses and ear protection.
- When piles are to be lifted, all precautions as prescribed in section 5.4 (lifting and hoisting) should be observed.
- There should be strict access restriction around the area of pile driving. There should be no concurrent operation at least within a radius equal to double the height of the pile driver.
- The hammer should be blocked at the bottom of the leads when a pile driver is not in use.

5.18 Diving Operations

The safety requirements of diving operations are as follows:

- People employed as divers should be between 20 and 55 years of age, and have adequate training under the supervision of an experienced diver.
- A diving team should consist of at least two divers, one signalman, one pump man and a qualified sailor (if the operation is being carried out from a boat). At every point in time during the diving operation, only one of the divers should be deployed while the second diver with a complete set of diving equipment should be available for deployment in emergency.
- People employed as divers should undergo pre-employment medical fitness screening and regular re-screening. No personnel who are indisposed should undertake diving operation.
- Safe means of access to and from the water, means of communication and lifeline with adequate belt should be provided to divers.
- Each diver should be provided with separate sets of warm clothing, woolens or flannels, woolen under suit, helmet and gloves.

- Breathing air supply compressor should have enough reserve to enable divers get to the surface and two emergency divers to and out of the diving depth if the equipment fails.
- The air supply line should be made of rubber reinforced with webbing, possess adequate breaking strength and be capable of withstanding the highest hydraulic pressure it will be subjected to without failing.
- Joints in the breathing air supply line should be by screw couplings.
- The air supply line should have: an air receiver; oil and water filters; a safety valve; a stop valve; a reducing valve; a pressure gauge; a carbon monoxide monitor. The elements in the oil and water filters should be changed at least every 3 months and the carbon monoxide calibrated annually.
- Diving equipment should be inspected, tested and found to be safe before being deployed for the first time. They should be re-inspected every three months.
- Air supply compressor, pump, cylinder and hose line should be tested for leakage prior to being used and re-tested every 24 hours.
- The inlet and outlet valves on the diver's dress and all regulator valves should be inspected within the past 24 hours and found to be functioning well before every operation.
- There should be a means of communication between the diver and the signal man. There should also be at least two means of communication between the diving team and emergency response personnel.
- When diving operation is in progress, appropriate signals should be flown at adequate distances (from all areas of approach to the location) to indicate that there are divers under water.
- Before the operation commences, the team should check the current condition, traffic, underwater pipes, cables and any other adjacent activity.
- When diving is to be done in dark places under water or in the night, there should be adequate and reliable means of lighting.
- Divers should not be deployed at depths exceeding 10 meters (33 feet) without authorization from a medical doctor.
- Before diving can be authorized at depths exceeding 10 meters (33 feet), there should be adequate compression and decompression facilities as prescribed by local regulations.

- There should be adequate first aid and rescue equipment as prescribed by local regulations or company standards during diving operations.

Underwater welding and flame cutting

- Only direct current should be used when carrying out under water arc welding.
- Equipment for underwater welding and flame cutting should be approved by local regulatory authorities.
- The underwater welder's PPEs should include insulated dress, helmet and gloves.
- The equipment should have a means of emergency shutdown that is accessible to the signalman.
- Electrode holders, electrodes, connections and conductors should be insulated with waterproof materials.
- Before electrodes are changed, the signalman should make the electrode holders dead and communicate the status to the welder.

Underwater blasting

- Explosives used for underwater blasting should be water proof and detonators should be the low-tension submarine type.
- Blasting cables, electric leads, connections and fuses should be adequately protected and insulated against the underwater conditions.
- Divers should be protected against the risk of objects striking against blasting equipment, dragging of leads and fuses, and entangling of the breathing air line in leads or fuses.
- Preparation of charges and attachment of detonators should be done on land or diving vessel.
- The blasting position should be clear from the surface of the water.
- Shots should be fired when the following conditions are met: the diver is out of the water; access restriction is effected from safe distances; every necessary precaution is in place; and the charge is re-checked to ensure it has not been displaced by water current.

5.19 Demolition Operations

Preparation for demolition

Before demolition operations start:

- The structure or facility should be adequately inspected and assessed for stability. Work should not begin until unstable parts of the structure are made safe or at least barricaded and sign posted.
- Power and utility lines should be safely disconnected. In the event that any of these is needed during the process of demolition, measures should be taken to protect and make it safe.

General requirements for demolition operations

- Demolition work should be carried out by personnel who have experience in such jobs. The operation should be supervised by very experienced and competent persons.
- The operation should start by the removal of loose objects, shutters and projecting parts of the structure.
- During the operation, workers should not be engaged in concurrent operations at different levels unless adequate measures have been taken to protect those at the lower levels.
- The operation should start from the top of the structure and go downwards.
- Demolished materials should not be allowed to accumulate so that the weight does not affect stability of the remaining structure.
- As the work progresses, regular assessment and care should be taken that parts that might affect the stability of the structure are not prematurely removed.
- During climatic conditions (like windy or rainy weather) that might affect the stability of the structure work should be suspended. Workers and equipment should be pulled out to safe locations until the condition improves.
- At the end of each shift or before going on break, the structure should be reassessed and ascertained that they are not in a condition that it

can be brought down by rain or wind. Otherwise, it should be propped up or fenced off and sign posted.

- To minimize dust, water should be sprayed as the demolition work progresses.
- If there is a wall, pillar or beam that is supporting a part of the structure, care should be taken not to demolish that supporting wall, pillar or beam until the part of the structure it is supporting has been removed.
- Safe access and egress should always be provided for workers on a demolition site.
- Workers in a demolition site should wear safety boots, hard hats, heavy gloves, safety glasses and appropriate respirators (if dust is being generated).
- When required catch platforms should be provided along the exterior walls of the structure being demolished so as to prevent danger from falling objects.

Demolition equipment

Due consideration should be given to the nature of a building or structure, its dimension, space from adjoining structures before determining the type of demolition equipment to use.

- If power shovels and bulldozers are to be used, the power of the equipment vis-à-vis the structure to demolish should be considered in addition.
- A safety zone having a width of 1.5 times the height of the structure should be maintained around the points of contact if a swinging weight is used.
- The weight should be controlled so that it does not dangle and cause damage to other structures not being demolished.
- Whichever equipment is used, it should be operated from a safe distance and no other worker should enter the safety zone except the operator.
- Scaffolds and ladders used should be independent of the structure to be demolished.

Demolition of structural steelwork, tall chimneys, and steeples

- Care should be taken to avoid the danger from any sudden twist, spring or collapse of structural steelwork when it is cut.
- Steelwork should be demolished tier by tier.
- Demolished steel parts should not be dropped from height but lowered gradually.
- Tall chimneys, steeples and such structures should not be demolished by blasting or overturning unless there is adequate space to take its dimension.
- When tall chimneys are to be demolished by hand, scaffolding should be used and it should be shifted as the operation progresses. Hoisting appliances should not be supported on the scaffold.
- If elevating work platform (EWP) is to be used care should be taken so that cut portions of the structure being demolished do not destabilize the EWP.
- Materials being removed can be thrown down inside the chimney provided there is an appropriate opening at the bottom for removal. And the materials should only be removed at break periods.

Appendix

LIST OF GENERIC HAZARDS

H-01 Hydrocarbons
- Crude oil under pressure
- Crude oil at low pressure
- Hydrocarbon gas
- NGL, Condensate
- Wax

H-02 Refined hydrocarbons
- Gasoline
- LPG
- LNG
- Kerosene
- Diesel (automotive gas oil)
- Low pour fuel oil
- High pour fuel oil

H-03 Other flammable products
- Wood, furniture & papers
- Flammable chemicals
- Dry grass
- Pyrophoric materials

H-04 Explosives
- Conventional explosive materials
- Detonators
- Explosive chemicals

H-05 Pressure hazards
- Bottled gas under pressure
- Water under pressure in pipelines
- Air under high pressure
- Reservoir pressure

H-06 Hazards associated with differences in height
- Personnel at height over 2m
- Overhead equipment
- Falling objects
- Lifting & hoisting

H-07 Objects under induced stress
- Objects under tension
- Objects under compression

H-08 Dynamic situation hazards
- Land transport (driving)
- Air transport (flying)
- Use of hazardous hand tools
- Use of hazardous power tools
- Equipment with moving or rotating parts

H-09 Environmental
- Heat stress
- Cold stress
- Avalanches
- Dust storm
- Wind, tornadoes, cyclones
- Flooding

- Lightning
- Landslide
- Earthquake

H-10 Hot surface
- Steam piping
- Process piping and equipment (temperature between 60 – 150 deg C)
- Process piping and equipment (temperature over 150 deg C)

H-11 Hot fluids
- Temperatures above 150 deg C

H-12 Open Flames
- Direct fired furnaces
- Welding
- Flame cutting

H-13 Electricity
- Voltage (50 – 440 volts)
- Voltage over 440 volts
- Static electricity

H-14 Electromagnetic radiation
- Elect radiation; high voltage ac cables
- Ultra violet radiation

H-15 Ionizing Radiation – open source
- Naturally occurring radioactive materials
- X-ray

H-16 Carcinogens
- Asbestos
- Other carcinogenic materials

H-17 Asphyxiates
- Excessive CO_2
- Insufficient O_2
- Other asphyxiates

H-18 Toxic gases
- Hydrogen sulfide, sour gas
- Chlorine
- Nitrogen oxides
- Other toxic gases

H-19 Toxic Liquids
- Miscellaneous chemicals (e.g. cleaning, pipeline, laboratory
- Mercury

H-20 Toxic solids
- Oil based sludge
- Calcium hydroxide
- Other toxic chemicals

H-21 Corrosive substances
- General acid dilutes
- Caustic soda
- Sulfuric acid
- Other corrosive chemicals

H-22 Biological
- Sewage (sanitary), virus and bacteria (water borne)
- Sexually transmitted disease
- Water borne bacteria (legionella)
- Insects, spiders, scorpions, bees
- Ebola
- Corona virus
- Other communicable diseases

H-23 Ergonomic Hazards
- Damaging Noise
- Manual material handling
- Awkward location of workplaces and materials
- Workstations
- Vibration
- Work planning issues

H-24 Psychological hazards
- Job security
- Work away from family
- Personal issues external to work
- Organization, system and culture

H-25 Security related
- Assault
- Theft/pilferage
- Armed conflict
- Terrorism
- Car jacking
- Kidnap
- Civil unrest
- Theft of sensitive information
- Organized crime

H-26 Work over water
- Boating
- Wading through water
- Work in swamp location
- Work offshore
- Transfer from boats to offshore locations
- Transfer from boat to boat
- Transfer from boat to swamp locations

H-27 Medical
- **Medical unfitness**
- **Lack of medical facilities**

H-28 Work in desert locations
- **Desert driving**
- **Desert survival**

H-29 Work in forest locations
- **Off-road driving**
- **Wild animals**
- **Snakes and dangerous reptiles**
- **Poisonous plants**

Printed in the United States
By Bookmasters